SUPARINPEI

ALSO BY

GILES HOPKINS

Wandering Along the Way of Okinawan Karate
The Kata and Bunkai of Goju-Ryu Karate

SUPARINPEI

The Last Kata of
Goju-Ryu Karate

GILES HOPKINS

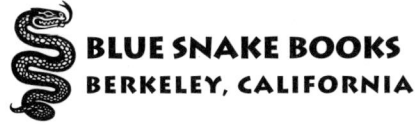

BLUE SNAKE BOOKS
BERKELEY, CALIFORNIA

Published by Blue Snake Books, an imprint of North Atlantic Books
Berkeley, California
Cover and interior photos by Jeff Cook
Cover design by Howie Severson
Book design by Happenstance Type-O-Rama

Printed in the United States of America

Suparinpei: The Last Kata of Goju-Ryu Karate is sponsored and published by the Society for the Study of Native Arts and Sciences (dba North Atlantic Books), an educational nonprofit based in Berkeley, California, that collaborates with partners to develop cross-cultural perspectives, nurture holistic views of art, science, the humanities, and healing, and seed personal and global transformation by publishing work on the relationship of body, spirit, and nature.

North Atlantic Books' publications are distributed to the US trade and internationally by Penguin Random House Publishers Services. For further information, visit our website at www .northatlanticbooks.com.

PLEASE NOTE: The creators and publishers of this book disclaim any liabilities for loss in connection with following any of the practices, exercises, and advice contained herein. To reduce the chance of injury or any other harm, the reader should consult a professional before undertaking this or any other martial arts, movement, meditative arts, health, or exercise program. The instructions and advice printed in this book are not in any way intended as a substitute for medical, mental, or emotional counseling with a licensed physician or healthcare provider.

Library of Congress Cataloging-in-Publication Data

Names: Hopkins, Giles, 1951– author.
Title: Suparinpei : the last kata of Goju-ryu Karate / Giles Hopkins.
Description: Berkeley, California : Blue Snake Books, 2021. | Includes index. | Summary: "An illustrated step-by-step guide to the structure, themes, and techniques of Suparinpei—the last kata of Goju-ryu. Suparinpei, or Pechurin, is the final and most difficult kata in the Goju-ryu system of Okinawan karate. Its performance has long been reserved for high-level practitioners, its history and applications obscured by misunderstanding and misinterpretation"—Provided by publisher.
Identifiers: LCCN 2020043118 (print) | LCCN 2020043119 (ebook) | ISBN 9781623175580 (Paperback) | ISBN 9781623175597 (ePub)
Subjects: LCSH: Karate—Japan—Okinawa Island. | Martial arts—Japan—Okinawa. | Hand-to-hand fighting, Oriental. | Suparinpei.
Classification: LCC GV1114.3 .H664 2021 (print) | LCC GV1114.3 (ebook) | DDC 796.815/30952294—dc23
LC record available at https://lccn.loc.gov/2020043118
LC ebook record available at https://lccn.loc.gov/2020043119

1 2 3 4 5 6 7 8 9 KPC 26 25 24 23 22 21

To Kimo sensei,
who first taught me Suparinpei

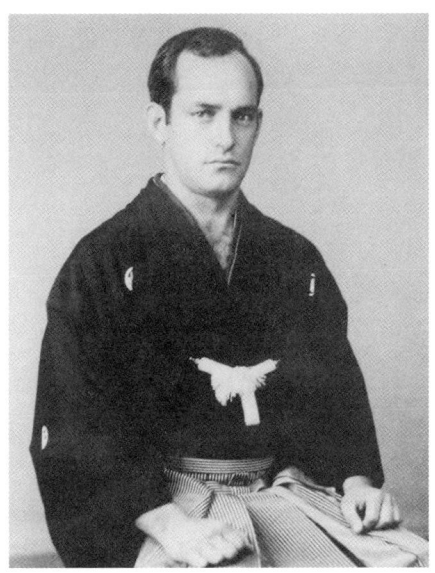

Kimo Wall sensei

ACKNOWLEDGMENTS

I WOULD LIKE TO EXTEND my thanks and appreciation to my teachers, Kimo Wall, Gibo Seiki, and Matayoshi Shinpo, and also to my indispensable training partner and friend, Bill Diggle.

I would also like to thank Jeff Cook, who took most of the photographs for this book, and my son, Noah, who assisted me with the two-person application photographs.

I want to thank the editors at Blue Snake Books for their help and patience with a difficult task, helping me to translate a movement art into words and pictures.

And lastly, of course, I would like to thank my family: Martha, Emily, Phoebe, and Noah. I couldn't do any of this without all of you.

CONTENTS

PREFACE

AFTER THE PUBLICATION OF MY first book, *The Kata and Bunkai of Goju-Ryu Karate,* someone suggested that it would have been better if I had illustrated *all* the techniques of *each* of the classical kata, but that book would have been thousands of pages long. This book is my compromise. I have tried to illustrate one complete kata here, Suparinpei, the last kata of Goju-ryu, and explain each of the applications. Of course, there are always constraints. No book, however well-intentioned, can take the place of a teacher. My intention in this book is not so much to teach the kata to someone who doesn't know it, but to shed light on a single enigmatic kata, and thereby, hopefully, deepen our collective understanding of Okinawan Goju-ryu karate.

Some years ago, I sat down to leaf through a book on T'ai Chi, where the author wrote what I think is a very telling summation of how many people nowadays approach kata and the martial arts in general. "I am not one of those teachers," he said, "who thinks that the actual physical movements of the form are to be used, as they stand, for self-defense."[1] Rather, he argued, we study the form in order to learn the principles. I think he is probably in good company. There are many practitioners of Okinawan karate, having long ago given up on the idea that kata can be deciphered or that these mysterious movements even have meaning in any martial sense, who subscribe to the notion that you can practice the skills and principles of kata without knowing how the movements were originally intended to be applied.

While it may be true, at least in a martial sense, that the aim of kata study is to understand the principles, it's certainly a stretch to imagine that we can discern the principles of any given system without first knowing how the seemingly arcane movements of kata were meant to be applied. The kata were created to preserve these principles of self-defense and teach them by showing examples of how to use them against an opponent. We can certainly practice generic principles, pound on the *makiwara* (punching post), and walk around the dojo holding the *nigiri game* (gripping jars), but the principles of any given system are contained within the applications of the techniques that are found in the kata or forms of that system. We can practice using the waist *(koshi)* or rooting or keeping the elbows down, but if we don't know how to use the techniques of the kata—how the techniques were originally meant to be applied—we won't understand why these things are important or why they are principles of the system we are practicing. Nor will we even begin to understand some of the principles that can only be grasped with a thorough understanding of the applications of kata. To imagine that we can learn the principles without knowing the applications seems to me as mistaken as putting the all too familiar cart before the horse.

It has always seemed a bit backward to me to suggest that the principles, or skills, as some refer to them, are the first things one should learn, only to be applied to the techniques of kata much later. How do you know that the principles you have come up with are the principles that derive from the system you are training unless you know how the techniques of that system are actually applied *(bunkai),* or to put it another way, how the movements of a given kata were originally meant to be used? And yet there are many that would say that it isn't possible to discover how the movements of kata were originally meant to be applied. The kata are too old and they were created too long ago, they say. Everything changes over time, and kata has no doubt changed too. But this is a rather pessimistic view, it seems to me. If we were simply to throw our hands up in resignation every time we encountered a puzzle, we might as well abandon science and bury our heads in the sandpile of discarded belief systems.

The problem, of course, may be that the kata themselves seem so impossibly incomprehensible. We know that the techniques are martial in nature, but we're not sure whether each individual technique is meant to be extracted and employed in *ippon kumite* (one point sparring) drills or whether we are meant to construct a kind of complementary shadow form to be used in a continuous two-person drill, as if we are reenacting a fight scene from a grade-B martial arts movie. There are even those who question whether kata was ever intended to be anything more than an exercise in focus and balance.

In fact, it seems to be a fairly widespread opinion even today, encapsulated in Patrick McCarthy's statement that kata is "a riddle, wrapped in a mystery, inside an enigma." As McCarthy noted twenty years ago, "the formula once used to interpret its [kata] application principles has all but vanished."[2]

And yet, ironically, at any large gathering of Okinawan karate practitioners—whether it's an annual *embukai* (show or public demonstration) or an instructional seminar—you are likely to see a number of performances of Suparinpei, particularly when there are high-level teachers in attendance. It almost seems as though it's expected that teachers of a certain rank, particularly those who have formed their own *kans* (schools), will demonstrate Suparinpei. I suspect that this is due in part to the hierarchical structure we use to teach Goju-ryu. The assumption is that Suparinpei, being the last and longest of the classical kata of Goju, is, therefore, the most difficult.

But we also assume, I think, that the mere performance of the solo kata, especially if it is by a high-ranking teacher, is somehow proof that the performer has mastered the system. We assume, in other words, that by watching only one side of an imagined confrontation—solo kata, after all, shows only the defender's actions—we can see not only how the techniques of the kata are meant to be used but how well the teacher uses them. It is difficult, however, to judge someone's understanding of the applications from a performance of the solo kata. Judging someone's understanding of a kata based on the snap of the uniform, or the perceived power of the punch, or how low the Horse Stance is, or, for that matter, any of the other rather nebulous criteria tournament judges might use at modern-day competitions, is superficial. At best, it is making judgments based solely on appearances, which, we know, can be deceiving. The punch that seems to be executed with power and precision may not be a punch at all, and may, in fact, require an entirely different kind of movement in application. Shouldn't the way we demonstrate kata reflect an understanding of its bunkai, its applications?

There are many, of course, that will dismiss this line of reasoning as mere pedantry. Kata, they say, can mean anything; that it is somehow limiting to suggest that the movements of kata were at one time meant to preserve specific applications. But how can we judge someone's performance of kata—and by inference their understanding of kata—if the interpretations of kata movements are just that, a matter of interpretation? Is it logical that kata were originally constructed to act as a generic template to provide an open-ended method for interpreting and applying technique? It seems much more plausible that the applications or bunkai of kata were at one time quite clear and specific and that the "formula once used to interpret" kata was somehow lost along the way.

This whole notion that the movements of kata can have multiple interpretations—what I would call "intentional ambiguity"—is hardly the most logical approach to kata. While this methodology may allow one to construct an effective martial art, accruing hundreds, if not thousands, of useful techniques, it's not a good way to unravel the principles or themes of a system, and ultimately, without any obvious organization, not a very good way to learn self-defense. In fact, I am sure it would rouse the ire and raise the hackles of that long-ago logician, William of Ockham. I suspect that a far more likely explanation is that without any understanding of how a kata is put together—that is, its structure and the fact that kata is composed of sequences, with each made up of receiving techniques, bridging techniques, and finishing techniques—people have tried to make sense of these seemingly esoteric movements with fearless abandon and endless invention. Following this inclination for creative interpretation, I would argue, is like wandering randomly in a dark forest; there is always the chance that we may discover something wonderful on our way through the woods, but more than likely we'll get lost somewhere along the way. Understanding the *structure* of a kata is one of the keys to understanding and interpreting the techniques and principles of the kata. And while there are always some things that may seem to be a bit ambiguous, this ambiguity, I believe, is not intentional.

If we don't consider the structure of the kata, and choose to ignore the foundation that logic and martial principles provide, then the applications we find—our interpretations of the movements of kata—generally fall into one or more of these categories: (1) those applications that don't follow the movements of kata; (2) those applications that aren't remotely realistic in any martial sense; (3) those applications that do not incapacitate the opponent, making him incapable of continuing or renewing the attack; and (4) those applications that do not take into account the themes the kata is exploring, so that they don't fit with the general tenor of the kata or the rest of the system.

One of the difficulties we encounter in this attempt to understand kata, however, is that the structures of the different classical kata vary—no two kata seeming to conform to exactly the same structure, as if there are no hard and fast rules of kata analysis.

For example, the structure of Seipai kata is fairly clear and straightforward, with five sequences. The first three are shown in their entirety only on one side, while the fourth and fifth sequences are shown on both sides, with a single finishing technique shown at the end of the kata. Kururunfa, on the other hand, begins with an opening or receiving technique on both the left and right sides followed by a finishing head twist shown three times. But unlike most of the other kata in the classical canon of Goju-ryu, the remaining three sequences of Kururunfa—the second and third sequences shown on both sides and the fourth shown only once—are meant to be attached to the opening Cat Stance techniques, or, at least, the position of the hands after the second of the Cat Stance kicks. That is, following the kicking techniques, the foot comes down into Basic Stance, with one hand palm-up at shoulder height and the other palm-down at about waist level. If we were to begin the kata from a grappling-like posture, the lower hand would have pushed down on the opponent's arm from the outside, and the upper hand would have come up inside the opponent's other arm from the inside. The implication is that each of the four sequences of Kururunfa begins with this same technique followed by the transitioning inside forearm technique that we also see in the second complete sequence of Suparinpei.

This is not really surprising, I suppose, since the origins of any of these kata belong to that proverbial mist-shrouded past. Even if these kata have all been collected under the rubric of Goju-ryu, we don't actually know whether they were originally part of the same system, only that they all share certain themes and methods of attack (or counterattack).

None of this would really matter since the present work is only concerned with Suparinpei kata, except that Suparinpei is not just thought to be another subject in the curriculum of Goju-ryu. Popular perception is that mastery of its movements, demonstrated through the solo kata performance, somehow denotes a mastery of the system. The supposition is that Suparinpei is somehow the embodiment of the principles and the techniques we find in all of the other kata.

Whether this is true or not is probably open to question since Suparinpei shows a *clear* relationship to only three of the other classical subjects of Goju-ryu—Sanchin, Sanseiru, and Seisan. And though it is hard to say whether it is the most difficult or the most technically complex kata, its structure may be the most challenging to unravel or really "see."

It's not exactly clear what purpose this structural opacity may have originally served. Was it used to intentionally hide the applications of the techniques? In the first half of the kata, we see the initial entry or receiving techniques—the *mawashi uke* (circular receiving technique) and *nukite/shuto* (spear hand or finger strike/knife hand strike)—separated from the three finishing techniques—the Cat Stance mawashi or *tora guchi* (a circular arm technique used to attack), the double punch, and the angular *shiko dachi* (Horse Stance) series. Each of these techniques is effectively *preserved* in the kata, which is after all the purpose of kata, and yet because they are not proximally connected—with the exception of the first mawashi in Cat Stance—it isn't immediately clear how they are meant to be applied. And yet we could say that nothing is really hidden. In fact, it would be easy to steal the kata—watching unobserved through a crevice in the garden wall—and still have no idea how the techniques were supposed to be used.

Or did the kata take on this form merely because it was the easiest shorthand method for preserving the techniques? If we go back to the kata and reintroduce the appropriate mawashi uke and nukite/shuto entry technique before each of the finishing techniques, and demonstrate both left and right sides, as some kata do, it certainly makes things clearer, but the kata becomes ungainly, needlessly long and repetitive, and, at least in a performance sense, rather clumsy. The first half of the kata is already quite repetitive. Perhaps the current iteration of Suparinpei—trying to imagine back to a time when there were only a number of techniques that may have been practiced in isolation—was compiled merely with an eye to its aesthetic balance.

The question of exactly *why* the structure of Suparinpei is so uniquely confusing is, of course, one of those questions whose answer is lost to time. We don't have written records that might help answer the more perplexing questions about kata, and certainly none that explain bunkai, the *Bubishi* notwithstanding. What we do have is the kata, passed on from teacher to student for generations.

Which all serves to remind me that many years ago now, I happened on a translation of the minutes of the 1936 meeting of karate masters, government officials, and journalists in Patrick McCarthy's *Ancient Okinawan Martial Arts: Koryu Uchinadi*. The meeting was sponsored by the Ryukyu Newspaper Company, but its primary organizer was Nakasone Genwa. Though Mr. Nakasone went on to publish a number of books on karate, he seemed a curious figure to be so instrumental in this gathering of prominent martial artists. The underlying agenda of the 1936 meeting—etched in fine print between the lines of text—was to find ways to popularize karate, make it more acceptable to the public, and give it a less violent image.

In his short essay titled "Karatedo Gaisetsu: An Outline of Karatedo," which McCarthy dates March 23, 1934, it is evident that Miyagi Chojun was already thinking about the nature of karate and its popular perception by the time of the 1936 meeting. In this early essay, Miyagi emphasized that "training in karate-do improves one's health" and that "physical and mental unity develops an indomitable spirit."[3] Certainly, these were laudable goals, and might even convince a wary public that the aim of true karate practice was to develop physical as well as spiritual strength—not, it would seem, to develop the ability to defend oneself or to employ lethal techniques in life-threatening situations.

The second order of business at the 1936 meeting, put forward by Vice Commander Fukushima Kitsuma of the regional military headquarters, was to recommend that new kata—Japanese kata with Japanese names— be created. The discussion is again couched in terms that suggest a need to popularize Okinawan karate, which, as Nakasone Genwa suggests, "is in a slump these days." However, in no uncertain terms, Miyagi says that "the classical kata must remain." In fact, he reiterates this point, under- lining the importance of the Toudi kata (the classical or *koryu* kata of Chinese origin) to an understanding of the art, saying, "classical kata must remain intact; otherwise they will be forgotten."[4]

We imagine this insistence, of course, was based on the belief that "secret principles of Goju-ryu exist in the kata," a quote often attributed to Miyagi. The quote, however, may be apocryphal; there is no way of knowing, though it is certainly something he may have believed. And the wonderful thing is that as long as the movements of the classical kata are preserved, the "secret principles" and in fact the original bunkai are there to be discovered.

My own thoughts on Suparinpei have changed and, I believe, matured over the years. My understanding now is different from the way I saw kata almost twenty years ago, when I first began writing about Goju-ryu for the *Journal of Asian Martial Arts*. The way I have come to see Suparin- pei has changed even since the publication of my first book, *The Kata and Bunkai of Goju-Ryu Karate*. Most of this, as I have tried to say here, is due to a better understanding of the structure of Suparinpei, how the kata is put together. Once one sees that structure, it's easy to see how the tech- niques are meant to be used, so much so that it seems a bit embarrassing, I often think, that I didn't see it sooner. But if Malcolm Gladwell is right and it takes ten thousand repetitions to master something, that's a lot of kata practice. Trudge off to training, put on a *gi*, sweat through basics, practice with the *hojo undo*, and then run through all of the classical kata a couple of times, not to mention training subjects like the Gekisai kata and any other peripheral subjects, and you may not even manage to do Suparinpei ten thousand times in a lifetime. And yet the old adage holds true: You must do the kata until the kata does you, as I was often told by my teacher, Kimo Wall sensei.

It is, understandably, a long journey. The teacher can only stand somewhere along the path and point the way, helping us avoid the pitfalls and the dead ends in an attempt to shorten the journey, encouraging us to keep going, because ultimately it is a journey of understanding that each of us must walk on our own.

1
INTRODUCTION TO SUPARINPEI

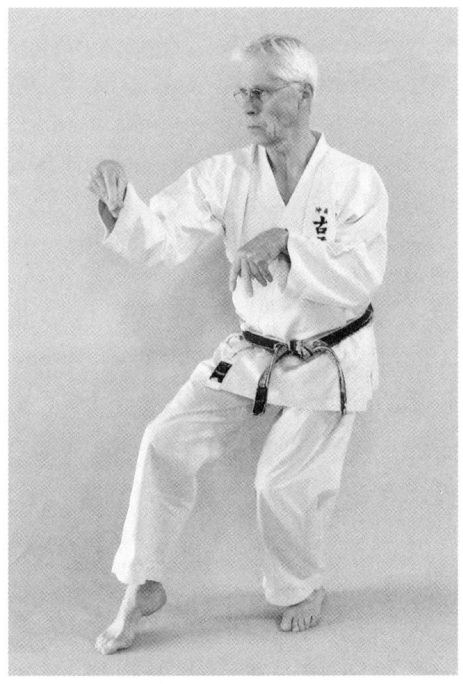

FIGURE 1.1 A variation of the final technique of the kata.

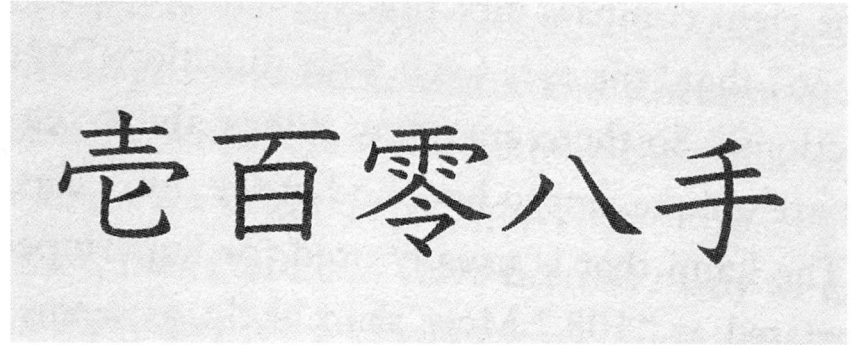

FIGURE 1.2 *Kanji* for Suparinpei.

THIS BOOK IS ABOUT SUPARINPEI, or Pechurin, as Matayoshi Shinpo sensei often referred to it, the last kata in the canon of Goju-ryu classical subjects. However, it is difficult to talk about any kata, even one as seemingly emblematic as Suparinpei, without touching on other kata, a method that may seem digressive, though perhaps unavoidably so if one is to really understand Suparinpei. Certainly there are subtle, and not so subtle, differences in how any of these kata are performed in different schools. It is my belief, however, that these differences are often merely idiosyncratic; whether we are discussing Sanseiru—the kata that exhibits the most differences among various schools—or Pechurin.[5]

The kanji that is usually used to designate the kata is generally translated as "108" or "108 hands." Though some have suggested that the name is merely a phonetic representation or Japanese pronunciation of the original Chinese name, the kanji itself has opened the door to all manner of speculation. For some, the character *te* (hand) at the end of the name suggests the number of techniques in the kata. But the notion that there are 108 techniques in Suparinpei most likely derives from the written form; the kanji for te written at the end of each kata name simply to remind the reader of the Chinese pronunciation, and more importantly, of the origin of the kata. In other words, the te character for "hand" may have little to do with the actual number of techniques we see in Suparinpei. For others, the name has long been thought to have Buddhist connotations, referring to the 108 mortal passions that plague mankind found in traditional Buddhist literature. The implication for the diligent karate-ka, of course, is that through the practice of this kata, one may overcome all of one's desires—desires, at least in the Buddhist sense, that bring suffering. More than any other kata, it seems to suggest a powerful connection between the physical practice of karate and spiritual enlightenment.

Even those who may be disinclined to attribute any spiritual significance to the practice of what was undoubtedly a brutal martial art may concede that the strict adherence to the movements of kata—whether one is practicing *chado* or *karatedo*—connects the mind and the body in a way that may remind some of that ancient Roman ideal of *mens sana in corpore sano* ("a sound mind in a sound body").

Some, on the other hand, have speculated that the name of the kata may simply be a reference, paying homage, in a way, to the legendary "Outlaws of the Marsh," the 108 bandit heroes depicted in the Chinese classic *Shui Hu Zhuan* (retold in English by Pearl S. Buck in her book *All Men Are Brothers*). This epic story, set in the ancient Song Dynasty, follows the exploits of a group of renegade warriors who try to right the wrongs they see around them.

Still others have suggested that the origin of the kata and its techniques may be traced to Yue Fei, a Chinese general who taught 108 empty hand fighting techniques that came to be called Yue Shi San Shou (Yue Fei's Fighting Techniques), eventually becoming the basis of Eagle Claw kung fu.

Of course, many of these stories are merely speculations about the significance of the name and there is no way of knowing the actual pedigree or historical authenticity of the kata itself. Oral tradition within some schools has suggested, unsubstantiated as it is, that there were originally three versions of Suparinpei—a *jodan* (upper level), *chudan* (middle level), and *gedan* (lower level) version—only one of which survives today, though it is unclear which of these possible versions the present-day kata represents. Some have suggested that only fragments of each are found within the present version.

Whatever the case, Suparinpei is the last kata taught in the canon of Goju-ryu classical subjects, and is, therefore, thought to be the highest embodiment of the principles and techniques of the system. This may be, however, more a matter of custom than any actual hierarchical structuring of kata or technique. Since each of the classical kata seems to explore a different theme, and the varied structure we find in each suggests disparate origins, a hierarchical arrangement based on a progression of difficulty or sophistication alone might be seen as completely arbitrary. However, since a large number of techniques in Suparinpei can be found in some form in the other kata of the system, there would seem to be some basis to argue that Suparinpei is a kind of compendium or perhaps summation of the techniques and martial strategies of Goju-ryu itself. At the very least, since Suparinpei is the longest kata in terms of actual movements, it is, I suppose, natural to assume that it is the most important and the most difficult to master.

Adding to the notion of Suparinpei's preeminent position is the oft-repeated suggestion that the other numerical kata—Seipai (18), Sanseiru (36), and Seisan (13)—are in some way lesser sisters of Suparinpei, if you will, because their numbers are each fractions of 108. This sort of search for meaning, however, falls flat fairly quickly. While 18 and 36 may be factors of 108, for whatever coincidental reason, 13 (Seisan) is clearly not—even though, for a number of reasons, the techniques of Seisan kata may be most closely related to Suparinpei. Furthermore, any attempt to count the number of techniques in any of these kata will not easily coincide with the number used to designate the kata, unless one is open to a fair amount of creative bookkeeping or imaginative number crunching.

In any case, speculation about the name and origins of Suparinpei and its place in the curriculum probably doesn't do much to help us understand the techniques of the kata or the principles of self-defense that these techniques illustrate.

When we consider the techniques themselves, there may be more reason to justify this sort of hierarchical ordering of kata. There would certainly seem to be at least a thematic component to the order of kata in the canon of Goju-ryu. The higher kata—Sanseiru, Seisan, Kururunfa, and Suparinpei—all deal with grappling or clinch scenarios or, perhaps more accurately, a close confrontation with both arms raised in front of the body.

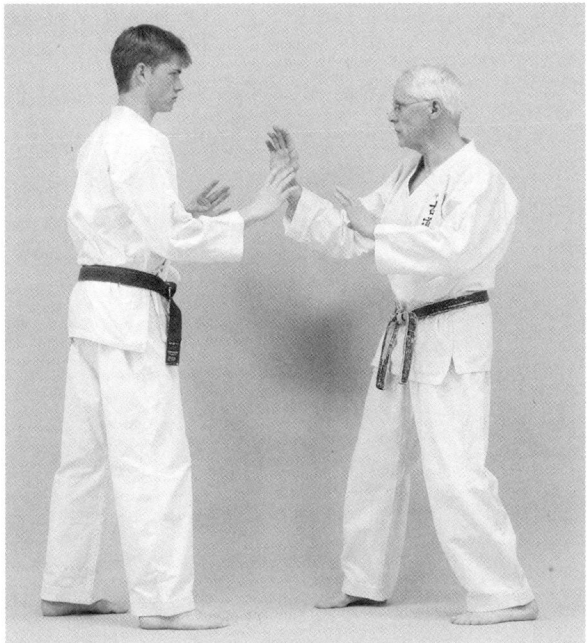

FIGURE 1.3 The scenario that we see in many of these kata begins with both arms raised in front of the body.

Three of these kata begin from this double-arm *kamae* (combat ready posture), suggesting that the opponent has also adopted this close-in fighting posture and that each of the entry techniques begins from this range. And, in fact, even in Kururunfa, though the kata does not begin in the double-arm kamae posture, the bunkai suggests that it too is showing techniques from a clinch or grappling position. In the first technique of Kururunfa, the defender's outside arm pushes in and down on the attacker's arm as the defender's inside arm is brought up to grasp the attacker's head. This is followed by a knee kick and down side kick.

In fact, oral tradition has always described Goju-ryu as a close-in martial style, which is why it often seems a bit counterintuitive to see demonstrations of Goju-ryu bunkai or ippon kumite characterized by long Front Stances and extended straight punches, reminiscent of the Gekisai kata, perhaps, or Shotokan, or even Tae Kwon Do, but not at all reflective of the techniques we see in the classical subjects of Goju-ryu. One could argue, from this standpoint, that this close-in range is a more challenging distance from which to engage an opponent—certainly more difficult to master—so that is why these kata are generally practiced later in the Goju-ryu curriculum.

Thematically, the earlier kata, particularly Saifa and Seiunchin, suggest simpler scenarios. The techniques of Saifa kata, for instance, seem to indicate that the bunkai sequences are a response to a same-side grab—that is, the opponent's left hand has grabbed the defender's right wrist or arm, for example, or vice versa.

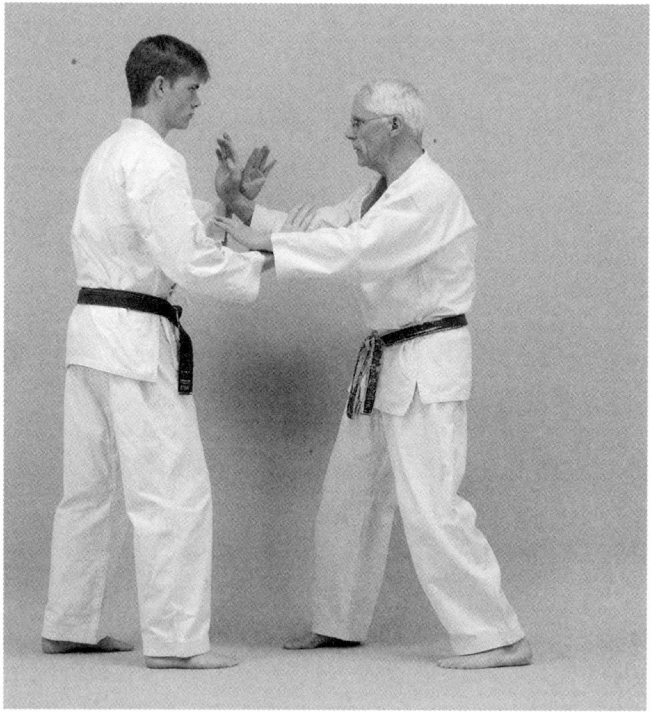

FIGURE 1.4 The classic starting posture we find in many close-combat martial systems, with one arm on the inside and one arm on the outside of the opponent's arms.

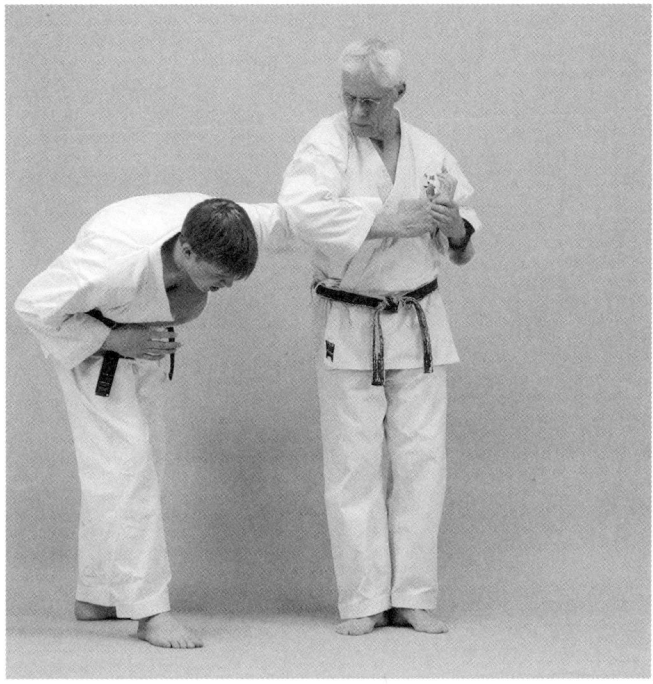

FIGURE 1.5 The first movement of Saifa kata responds to a same-side wrist grab by bringing the elbow and forearm over the attacker's arm.

Each of the five bunkai sequences of Seiunchin kata (not counting repetitions) is a response to a cross-hand grab—that is, the opponent's left hand, for example, has grabbed the defender's left wrist or arm—or a two-handed push. Though some have suggested that these sorts of wrist grabs are unlikely to occur in a real confrontation, this bias or skepticism comes largely from the notion that a realistic confrontation somehow mimics what we generally see in *jiyu kumite* (free sparring) contests at a karate tournament. In a real confrontation, where grappling is likely to occur, it is highly likely that one would attempt to grab and control the opponent's wrist or arm. Saifa kata shows how to deal with a same-side wrist grab, or what we see in the application of each of the entry techniques for the three sequences of the second half of Suparinpei kata (see figs. 2.66–67). In each of these sequences, the defender has moved inside the opponent's clinch to block and grab the attacker's right arm with his or her left hand, while counterattacking with the right hand. Seiunchin kata shows how to deal with a cross-hand wrist grab, or what we see in the application of the mawashi uke in the opening section of Suparinpei kata (see fig. 2.13).

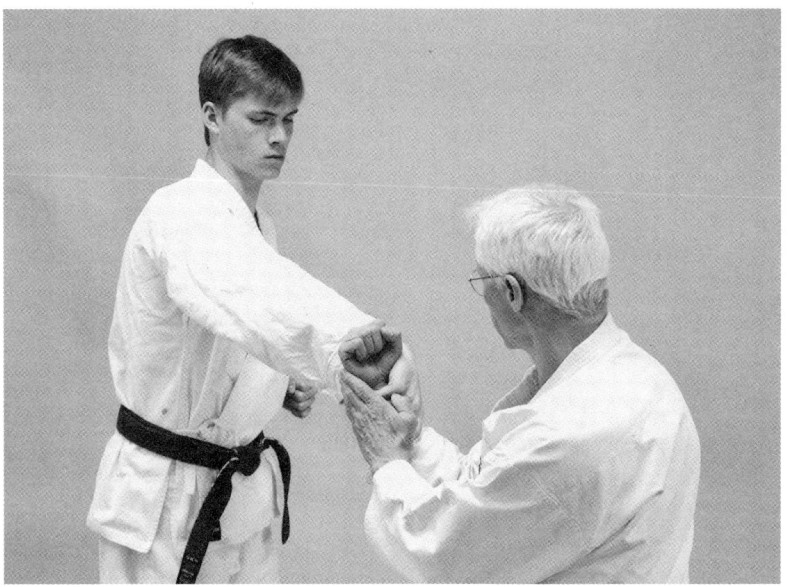

FIGURE 1.6 The second sequence of Seiunchin begins by trapping the hand of the opponent who has grabbed the defender's right wrist.

This perspective—looking at the opponent's method of attack—may be some rationale for the order of kata, the hierarchy, or it may just be a rationalization to explain and justify the order we have put the kata in, though that order is by no means universal. In fact, the techniques of Shisochin kata also seem to illustrate responses to an attack where the opponent has used both arms, another way of describing the grappling scenario.

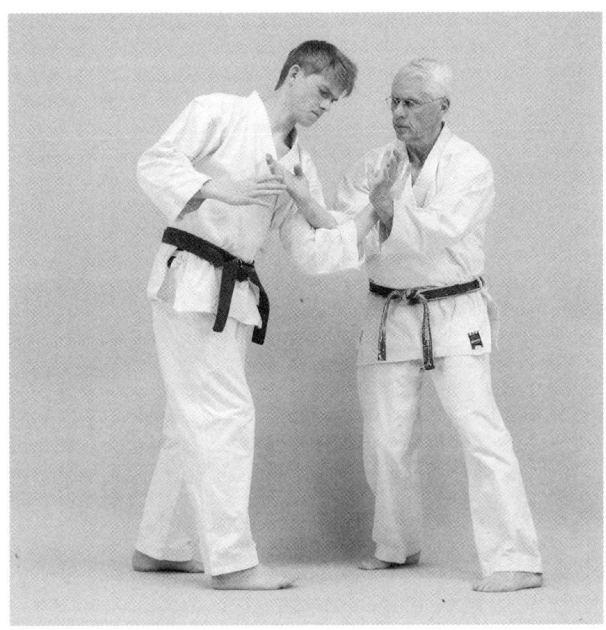

FIGURE 1.7 Pivoting into the opening posture of Shisochin from a clinch brings the attacker's head forward and down.

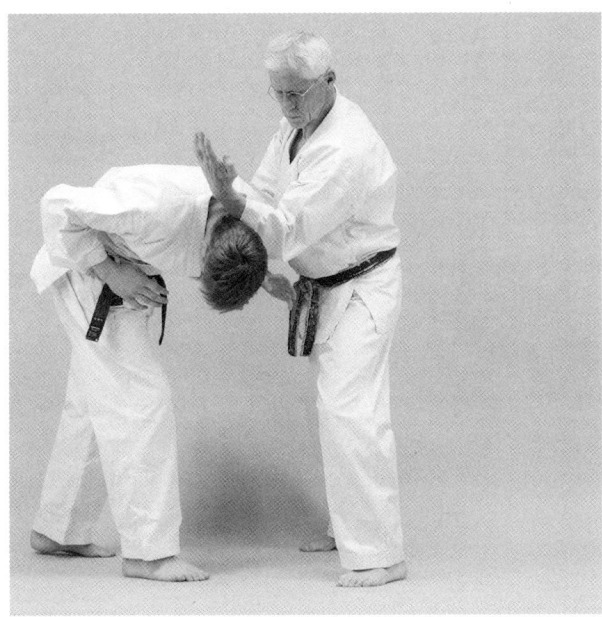

FIGURE 1.8 Stepping in with the forearm angle technique, in this variation, controls the opponent's head. This sequence continues with a forearm attack and head-twisting technique.

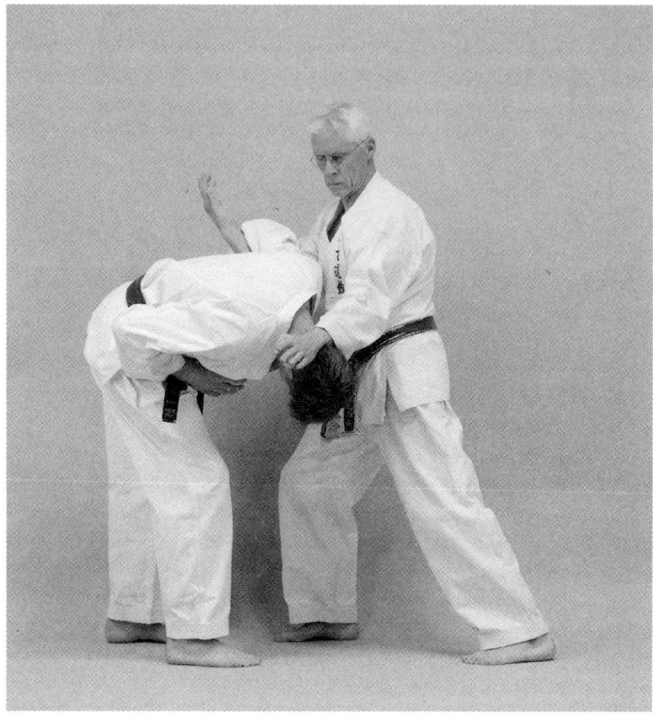

FIGURE 1.9 This second method of using the forearm angle
technique from Shisochin is also used to control the opponent's
head, and seems to be the more likely application. We generally
see one or the other of these techniques in the demonstration
of kata from different Okinawan Goju-ryu schools. In the first
of these angle techniques, the kata practitioner's line of sight
is directed forward to the right hand. In the second, the practitioner is focused on the lower left hand.

And though the techniques of Seipai kata seem to be particularly
effective against a single-hand lapel grab, it is admittedly difficult to
be sure, as the initial receiving techniques work equally well against a
punch, two-handed lapel grabs, or the clinch/grapple scenario, suggesting at the very least that we may see responses to each type of attack in
this kata.

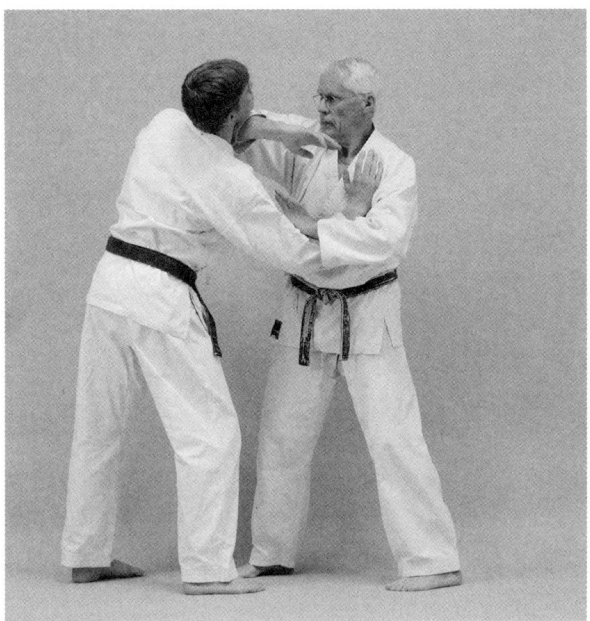

FIGURE 1.10 In response to a lapel grab, the defender's left arm is brought down on the arm of the attacker as the right elbow is brought up to attack the opponent's head in the opening technique of Seipai kata. Then the right arm straightens out to bring the opponent's head down as the sequence continues.

About the only thing different schools can agree on is that Saifa is where our practice of the classical Kaishu kata usually begins and Suparinpei is at the end. In one sense, we could argue that any order is completely arbitrary and reflects no more than a personal bias since each kata presents its own unique scenarios, which is as it should be; there is little need for redundancy in a martial system.

The use of the term *kaishu* (open-hand) kata to refer to the eight classical kata is somewhat perplexing in itself. Suparinpei, Seisan, and Sanseiru all begin with a closed-fist double-arm kamae. The initial movements of each kata are thought to represent either slow or fast punches. And in both Seisan and Sanseiru there are additional punching-like techniques. While I have always thought that most of these "punches"—if not all of them—really only indicate that the defender has grabbed the opponent, wouldn't grabbing, pulling, and twisting techniques be clearer in the Kaishu kata if all of the techniques that utilized a grab were shown as open-hand techniques? If, as legend suggests, Miyagi sensei closed the hand in Sanchin kata, perhaps Sanseiru and Seisan and Suparinpei also originally began with open-hand techniques.

Some have suggested that Suparinpei is always the final kata in the canon of Goju-ryu classical subjects because it serves as the embodiment of all the techniques and principles one has encountered in the practice of all the other classical subjects—that every technique we see in each of the other kata can be found in Suparinpei, only here they are practiced on a higher level. At the very least, however, these statements are a bit misleading. Certainly one will naturally incorporate everything one has learned in the way of principles or movement by the time one learns Suparinpei. But it is a bit of unsubstantiated hyperbole to suggest that Suparinpei contains *all* of the techniques of the other kata. We certainly see the techniques of Sanchin in Suparinpei, which is understandable, but for the most part, as far as the Kaishu kata are concerned, Suparinpei shows only a marked similarity to the techniques of Sanseiru and Seisan. Most of the other classical subjects show only a few coincidental similarities. This suggests that there may be a similar origin to these four kata—Sanchin, Sanseiru, Seisan, and Suparinpei—and that the other classical kata, though they may be part of the same system as some common themes and principles would suggest, were added later or came from a different source.

This, of course, is merely speculation and falls in that pile of unanswerable questions we inevitably accumulate as we look to understand the message of kata. Since there really are no actual written records—notwithstanding the few technical sketches we have from the *Bubishi*—we need to rely heavily on guesswork, which to many seems to be a license to interpret kata movements in any way that seems to remotely replicate kata, with even further latitude to wander from a strict interpretation of

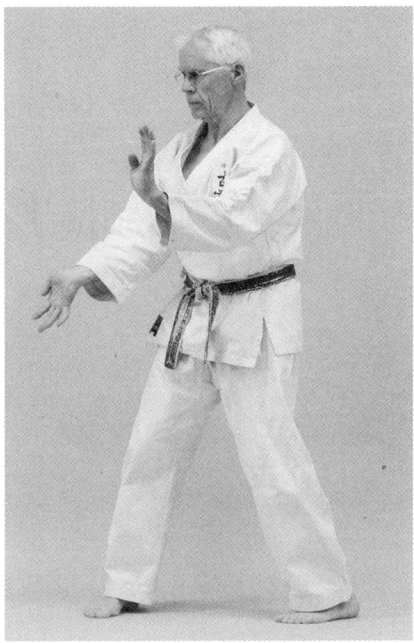

FIGURE 1.11 The mawashi uke in
sanchin dachi (Basic Stance) only occurs
in Sanchin, Tensho, and Suparinpei.

the movements of kata when we employ terms such as *henka bunkai* or
oyo bunkai. But guesswork is merely formulating a hypothesis, much as
we would do if we were attempting to explain things we didn't understand
in the world around us. If we were employing the scientific method, we
would formulate a hypothesis and, using an experiment, test the hypothesis, making sure that it also conformed to the laws of nature. This last
point corresponds to good martial principles and logic. In the case of kata
and bunkai, in other words, we should ask whether our explanation of
kata and kata technique reflects an understanding of good martial principles, and, at the same time, whether the bunkai is realistic as we test it out
in some form of *kumite*.

Some, of course, balk at the idea that anyone today, this far removed
from the early days of karate or still further removed from the murky

past when these forms and kata were first created, can determine the original intent of kata, or more specifically how the movements of kata were originally intended to be used. They may be right; we can only make a best guess. But isn't this what we are all looking for, even when the task seems ultimately inconclusive, or the "answers," at best, seem ambiguous? And, after all, a study of the bunkai or techniques of kata reveals the martial principles upon which the system itself is rooted. We don't have any written records to validate our conclusions. The illustrations we see in the *Bubishi* show techniques that seem to come from a variety of different martial traditions. We can find techniques from Suparinpei and Kururunfa, but we also see illustrations that seem to be depicting techniques from Uechi-ryu kata or Shorin-ryu kata. And in any case, the techniques are merely fragments, small pieces of a sequence of kata movements. We don't, in fact, see anything more than snapshots of an encounter, with one or the other of the participants in an advantageous position. Should we rely on an ancient sampling of sketches whose origins are as cloudy as the origins of the kata themselves? Perhaps the *Bubishi* was merely a collection of musings or marginal doodles by someone who was also trying to figure out what these movements meant.

Can we find the original intent of kata, any kata, not just Suparinpei? Can we *reverse engineer* these seemingly arcane solo movements to get at a series of techniques that both illustrate very specific self-defense scenarios and teach the principles of this particular martial system?

Personally, I don't believe it's logical that someone long ago purposely created *generic* movements that could each be interpreted and applied in a variety of different ways, limited in many cases only by the practitioner's imagination. I know that there are many, however, who subscribe to this notion, whether out of frustration or simply because kata presents itself as a seemingly inexhaustible playground. After all, we are often told that the study of karate is a lifetime endeavor. If each kata were an encyclopedic collection of techniques, however, we would have considerable difficulty using *any* of the techniques we see in the kata in real confrontations or situations where we might need to draw on what we know to defend ourselves. What we draw on in these kinds of situations, of course, are the principles of movement that we have learned from kata, practiced until they are incorporated into "muscle memory," and tested in drills in the dojo. It is these principles that help to clarify our interpretation of the techniques of kata. And because they are all based on the same principles, the classical kata show a limited number of techniques, which, in many ways, show variations on a limited number of themes. In fact, a good explanation of kata will show how the movements of any one kata reinforce our understanding of all the other kata—a way that we can understand Goju-ryu as a system.

In other words, we should be able to see the same principles throughout the system. Some principles may be particular to particular systems, but other principles are common to most martial systems regardless of where they originated. One of these common principles, for example, is the notion that the elbow should drop or be kept down. We see this in the initial double-arm posture of Sanchin and Suparinpei kata. The techniques or self-defense scenarios of kata, however, help to illustrate the necessity of this principle. For example, in dealing with the opponent's wrist grab from the first sequence of Seiunchin kata, one discovers fairly quickly that it is much easier to release the opponent's grip and ultimately control the confrontation by dropping the elbow and rotating the arm, while stepping out toward the opponent, at an angle, into shiko dachi. In the subsequent moves of this sequence from Seiunchin kata, the defender controls the attacker's arm in such a way that the opponent is not given the opportunity to continue the attack (another principle), bringing the head down for the counterattack. And this, too, the idea that we block the arms but attack the head, is also one of the principles we see in Goju-ryu. The predominance of middle-level techniques in kata—and this would include punches—is because the opponent's head has been brought down to this level with the previous techniques of the sequence. This, in turn, is another reason it is important to identify the application sequences in any given kata.

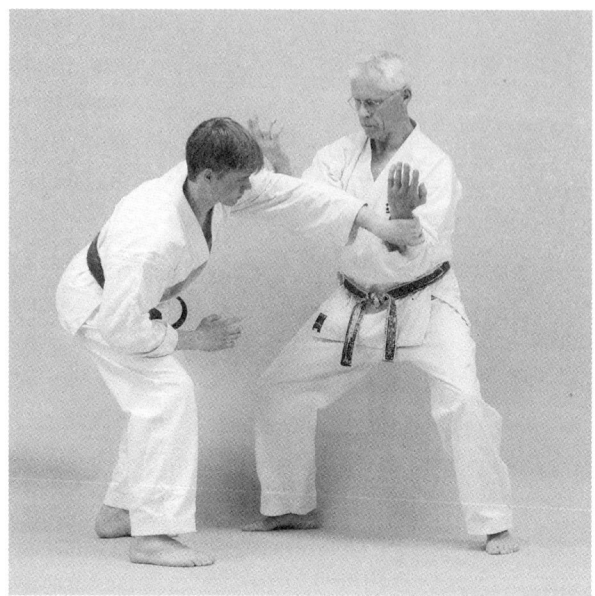

FIGURE 1.12 Dropping the elbow from the first technique in Seiunchin kata.

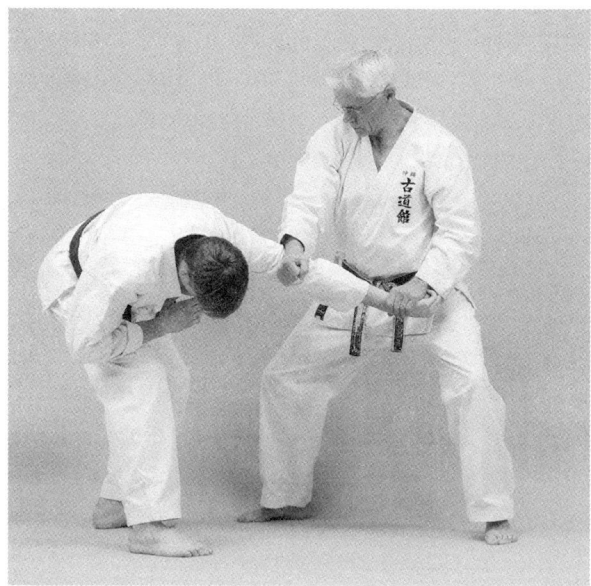

FIGURE 1.13 The second movement from Seiunchin kata controls the opponent's arm and brings the head down.

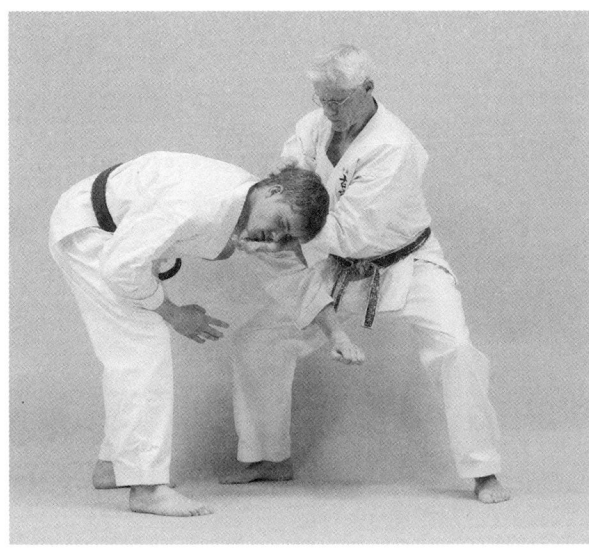

FIGURE 1.14 The third movement in Seiunchin kata is used to grab and attack the opponent's head.

But the idea that Suparinpei contains all of the techniques of each of the other kata is certainly a bit of fanciful thinking, serving only to feed the mystical notion that Suparinpei is a sort of umbrella kata, blanketing the system like the ten thousand stars in the heavens of ancient Chinese cosmology.

This notion may spring from the number of movements that make up the kata, but it may also, in part, arise from its structure; the structure of Suparinpei is not quite like any of the other kata. While each of the Kaishu kata is unique, there are enough similarities of structure that, for the most part, they seem fairly easy to decipher given certain common "rules." Suparinpei, on the other hand, seems confusing, at least initially, because the first half of the kata comprises incomplete sequences or sets of individual techniques taken out of context, as it were. For example, the double punch–right arm parry–left middle-level punch combination that is repeated four times doesn't begin with an entry or receiving *(uke)* technique, which has prompted many practitioners to take it at face value, suggesting that it is nothing more than a double punch or *awase tsuki* to the opponent's torso.

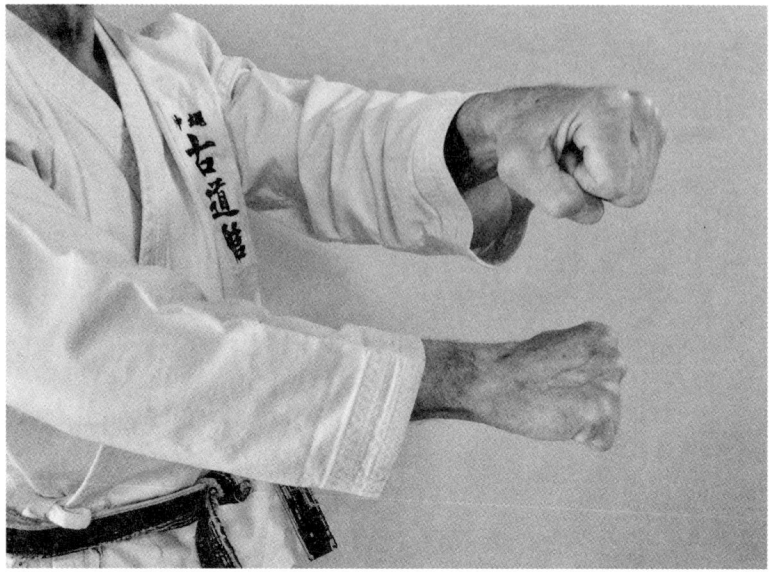

FIGURE 1.15 The double punch–right arm parry–left middle-level punch combination in Suparinpei kata is one of the finishing techniques that comes off the initial mawashi uke–tora guchi entry technique.

Additionally, none of the other classical kata repeat techniques four times, so there is no other reference point to help determine the "message" of that aspect of the kata. In Seiunchin there are four "elbow" techniques in Cat Stance, but they are meant to be applied in pairs. Shisochin kata, with its four forearm angle "blocks," may be the exception, though even there the repetition may, in fact, be an indication that two of the four techniques are showing a variation in application.

Three of the other Kaishu kata—Saifa, Seiunchin, and Seipai—begin with more or less complete bunkai sequences, while Shisochin and Sanseiru differ only in that three "nukite" (Shisochin) and *"tsuki"* (Sanseiru) techniques are tacked onto the beginning. (Convention suggests that the three opening techniques of Shisochin are nukite—that is, finger or spear-hand strikes. However, it is just as likely that these "nukite" techniques are really palm-heel strikes *(shotei)* or even scissoring techniques done with the forearms. The slow "punching" techniques that we see at the beginning of Sanseiru kata should probably be thought of as scissoring or arm-folding techniques, given the nature of the bunkai that we see in the sequences of the kata, rather than "tsuki" or punching attacks.) The opening structures of kata become a bit more complex with the last three Kaishu kata—Seisan, Kururunfa, and Suparinpei.

There are other differences as well. The five sequences of Seiunchin kata are fairly balanced, with the same sequences of techniques repeated on both the right and left sides (except for the finishing techniques of the first and fifth sequences).[6] This is probably an important consideration for single wrist grab attacks; it's useful to practice these techniques against a right wrist grab or a left wrist grab. But kata like Seisan or Sanseiru or Suparinpei are mostly one sided, which may have more to do with the fact that they begin from the double-arm kamae posture and what that implies.

And at least Seisan kata—somewhat similar to Suparinpei—begins with what seems to be a series of three sets of "basic" techniques, followed by three complete bunkai sequences. This is similar to what we see in the first half of Suparinpei, with its collection of partial sequences, followed again by three complete bunkai sequences. This is only confusing, however, because the first half of the kata is disjointed; the techniques are not strung together in a contiguous, complete bunkai sequence, with an entry technique, a controlling or bridging technique, and a finishing technique the way techniques are shown in the second half of the kata. Interestingly, the mawashi uke, fundamental to both Sanchin and Suparinpei, seems to be the key to understanding this structure. And understanding the structure of a kata is the key, I would argue, to understanding the techniques themselves.

Finally, I think, it is important to understand Suparinpei, the last kata one usually encounters in the practice of Goju-ryu, because Suparinpei, ironically, helps us understand so much else about the system. Since Suparinpei kata has disconnected techniques strung together (what we see in the first half of the kata) and longer sequences of techniques (what we see in the second half of the kata), it reinforces not only the notion that the techniques of each of the Kaishu kata compose sequences of entry techniques, bridging or controlling techniques, and finishing techniques, but also the idea that certain techniques may be taken apart and reassembled to show variations—something we see in the first half of the kata, where the mawashi uke serves as the entry technique for the three finishing techniques that follow it.

But Suparinpei also helps to explain Sanseiru and Seisan. It is Suparinpei that contains both the two-arm scissoring entry technique of Sanseiru (and Shisochin) and the "sun and moon" entry technique of Seisan, two of the three entry techniques shown in Suparinpei. And, of course, there are other similarities one may find in Suparinpei, not just to Sanseiru and Seisan, but to many of the other Kaishu kata as well. Suparinpei, in fact, is the key, I believe, to really understanding Goju-ryu.

2

The Techniques of Suparinpei

The Beginning Posture *(Yoi)*

See figures 3.1–4.

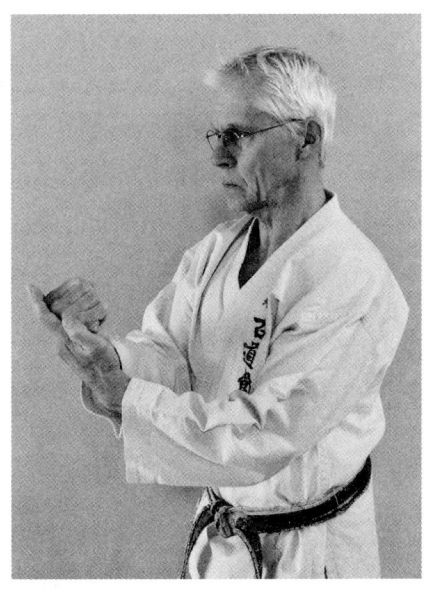

FIGURE 2.1 The beginning posture (yoi).

THE KATA BEGINS IN WHAT is referred to as *musubi dachi,* the body straight with the heels together and the feet pointed out at an angle. The hands are then brought together and up in front of the chest as the breath is drawn in, with the palms facing in, the left palm pressing against the back of the right hand. The hands are then rotated and lowered, still pressed together, until they are brought to a position out in front of the waist. As the hands are lowered, the breath is slowly exhaled, and the mind is focused on the *dantian* or *tanden.* Then the hands and feet separate, the hands closing into fists at the sides and the feet opening into *heiko dachi* (Parallel Stance), at the width of the shoulders. In some schools, the right hand closes into a fist as the hands are brought up in front of the body and then opened again when the hands reach the lowered position, or the right hand remains closed as the left hand closes with the separation of the hands and feet. In any case, these movements are more preparatory in nature.

This formal beginning to Suparinpei kata is shared by all of the classical Goju-ryu subjects. It is a formality, without the martial intent that we see in the movements of the rest of the kata, but it should not be dispensed with or treated as if it were entirely empty of meaning. The purpose here is to focus one's attention and breath prior to beginning the kata.

The Double-Arm *Kamae* Posture and Punches

See figures 3.5–15.

Once the attention is focused, the mind is calm, the breath is settled, and balance has been achieved with the practitioner standing in heiko dachi, the kata begins with a step into a right-foot-forward sanchin dachi with both arms brought up into the familiar double-arm kamae posture. This is the same posture that begins Sanchin, Sanseiru, and Seisan. How one brings the arms up into this posture may, in fact, be quite significant, depending on how one interprets this posture and the position of the arms—whether these three steps and "punches" are, in fact, techniques with real application or merely an exercise in practicing fundamental coordination of the arms and the breath along with proper posture and alignment. Some schools will raise the arms together in two sweeping arcs, while other schools will bring both arms up alongside the ribs and then circle out. And still others will bring one arm up and then the other. If the final position of this kamae, however, is simply meant to indicate the distance and posture one adopts in a grappling or clinch scenario, then it makes little difference how the arms are brought up. What is important is the angle of the arms and the position of the elbows, like Sanchin.

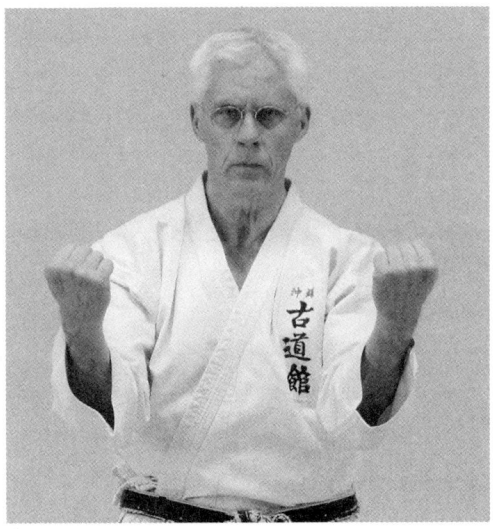

FIGURE 2.2 The double-arm kamae posture that begins Sanchin, Sanseiru, and Suparinpei.

Structurally, Suparinpei is probably most like Seisan kata in that the complete bunkai sequences—techniques that are strung together with an entry technique, a bridging or controlling technique, and a finishing technique—occur primarily in the second half of the kata. The kata begins with three slow "punches" in sanchin dachi executed from the double-arm kamae posture, similar to Sanseiru. These closed-fist techniques, of course, also resemble the slow punches in Sanchin kata. In Seisan kata, on the other hand, the beginning punches executed from sanchin dachi are fast.

It would be fair to ask why the punches are done slowly, often with a good deal of dynamic tension, sometimes accompanied by the contraction of what seems like every muscle in the body as the punch reaches full extension. In the case of Sanchin, a *kihon* kata, one might argue that all of the techniques of the kata are foundational; that is, Sanchin practice, done slowly and with deliberation, affords one the opportunity to focus on posture, breathing, stance, skeletal alignment, and all of those fundamental things that underlie the proper execution of any technique.

But there are very few actual techniques in Sanchin kata—a "punch," a palm-up and palm-down blocking or parrying technique, what appears to be a grab and pulling-in technique, and a mawashi technique in Basic Stance. Each of these techniques occurs in either Seisan or Suparinpei. In other words, with the exception of Seisan and Suparinpei, it would seem to be a rather weak argument to suggest that the few techniques we find in Sanchin kata actually provide the foundation for the rest of the Goju-ryu system. Certainly there are fundamental principles of movement and structure that Sanchin practice serves to instill in the student. But the techniques themselves do not necessarily help us understand the techniques we find in most of the other classical subjects.

Still, there is something fundamental here. What these four kata share—Sanchin, Sanseiru, Seisan, and Suparinpei—is that they begin in Basic Stance with both arms held up in front of the body. Oral history tells us that at one time, the Sanchin kata of Goju-ryu was an open-hand kata; that Miyagi Chojun sensei closed the hands. If this is indeed true, it might suggest that the "punches" we see at the beginning of these kata, particularly the slow punches, may have been more about pushing and pulling to unbalance an opponent than about middle-level percussive attacks. This idea that the first step in dealing with an opponent—prior to the application of any of the techniques we see in the bunkai sequences of these kata—is to push or pull them to destroy their balance is certainly one that makes sense. And it matters little whether you choose to illustrate this with open hands or closed hands. Perhaps to Miyagi sensei, the closed hand encouraged the student to work on grip strength and illustrated grabbing the opponent. We can only guess, but it seems like a logical explanation given the nature of the techniques we see in these kata.

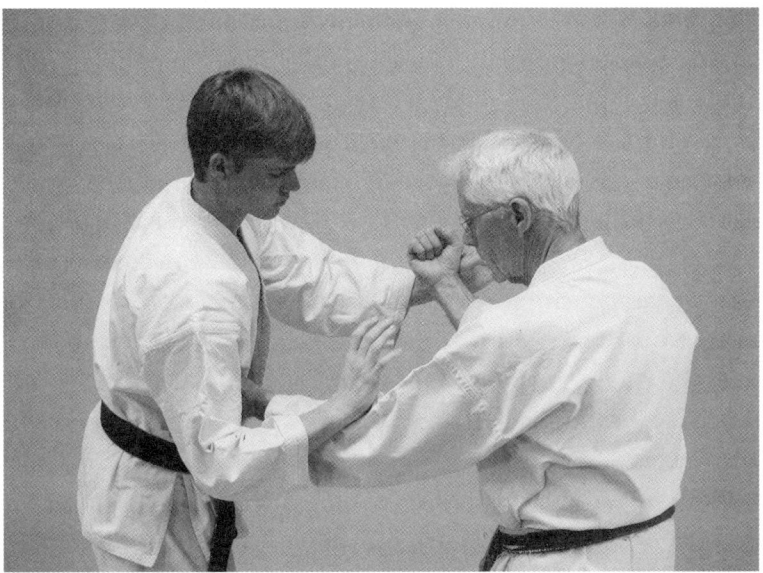

FIGURE 2.3 The slow "punches" may be intended to mimic the pushing action used to upset the opponent's balance.

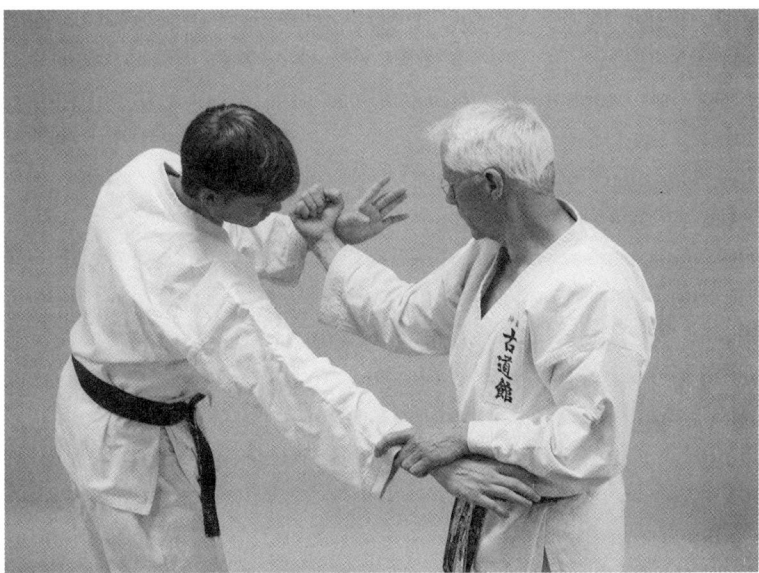

FIGURE 2.4 The retraction of the "punch" mimics the pulling action used to upset the opponent's balance.

If that is indeed the case, then one should also probably question the execution of the slow "punches." Certainly all of the traditional principles should apply, whether one is actually punching or pushing—the elbow should be kept down and the arm should move in and out along the side of the body or ribs. But what we see so often in the execution of Sanchin (or the opening of Suparinpei) is that the focus seems to be on the rigidity of the body, as if the student is emulating the rooted sturdiness of an oak tree. The only thing that moves—once the student settles into this opening right-foot-forward posture or steps into the next left-foot-forward posture—is the right or left arm, slowly retracted and slowly pushed out until the arm is fully extended, and then once again pulled back into the double-arm kamae posture. In other words, there doesn't seem to be any use of koshi ("the waist"); nothing moves but the arm, and even that often seems to be struggling against the student's use of dynamic tension, as if it's not clear whether the arm should be held back or pushed out.

Yet it is widely believed that one of the most important aspects of any martial technique is the use of koshi. And while it may be desirable to practice a well-rooted stance (though I think *balance* may be a more accurate term to use here), the subtle movement of the upper body, including the waist, I believe, is an important part of these opening techniques. It is the waist, after all, that moves the arms, whether they are extending or retracting, pushing or pulling, punching or blocking. The focus should be on the movement of the trunk of the body, the student's core, pivoting around the spine, from the waist to the shoulders, however subtle that movement may appear as it is developed over time and practice.

Beyond that, however, there is a difference, one might imagine, between the practice of what appear to be fundamental techniques in Sanchin kata, one of the Heishu or kihon kata, and Kaishu kata like Suparinpei. In the practice of Sanchin, as Miyagi Chojun sensei says in his 1934 short essay titled "Karatedo Gaisetsu: An Outline of Karatedo," "students learn to regulate their breath while coordinating it with the use of their power in a correct posture" in order to "[cultivate] a strong physique while encouraging a *budo* spirit." In Kaishu kata like Suparinpei, we are practicing specific "offensive and defensive techniques," as Miyagi says, shown in various self-defense scenarios.[7]

That being said, it is not only tempting but, I would suggest, highly likely that these slow "punches" at the beginning of Suparinpei may be different in intent from the slow punches we see in Sanchin kata. In Sanseiru we see the same set of three "punches" executed in Basic Stance, stepping forward with a double-arm kamae, where the "punch" and its retraction into the double-arm posture serves as the initial entry technique for each of the sequences that are practiced later in the kata.

Starting in a clinch posture with both arms up (see fig. 1.4), with one arm on the outside of the opponent's arm and one arm on the inside, a posture similar to what one might see in a typical wrestling match or Okinawan sumo contest, the defender simply pivots in response to the opponent's inside arm thrust, whether that attack is a punch, a push, or

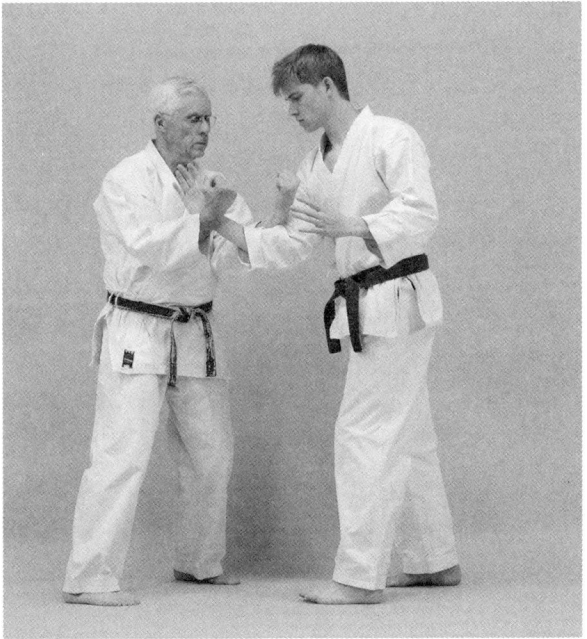

FIGURE 2.5 The double-arm kamae used as an entry technique in Sanseiru kata. As the opponent attacks with his or her right arm, the defender pivots, pushing against the outside of the attacker's arm while bringing the other arm up inside the attacker's arm.

a reaching grab. The defender's outside arm pushes against the attacker's arm as the defender's inside arm pulls in against the attacker's arm. This scissoring action of the two arms effectively turns the attacker and begins to bring the attacker's head down to continue the counterattack. In the case of Sanseiru, the kata shows three methods or examples of how to bridge or move in on the opponent after executing this scissoring or arm-folding technique.

In Suparinpei it is certainly likely that the kata is showing a similar technique or method of dealing with a grappling kind of confrontation with the opponent rather than simply executing slow punches in order to practice the coordination of the body and breath or proper posture, something one would hope to have mastered by the time one took up the practice of Suparinpei. Kata, after all, is the physical record of theme-related self-defense applications—there is no need to incorporate practice drills within the confines of a Kaishu kata, with its limited number of moves. This double-arm kamae with its "punch" and retraction is, therefore, more likely the first of three different receiving or entry techniques in Suparinpei.

The slowness of the "punches," then, along with the awareness that one is really using the entire body, is meant to focus one's attention, I suspect, on the pushing and pulling nature of these techniques. We practice them slowly not to learn proper punching alignment but to mimic the movements of pushing and pulling an opponent in order to break their balance, employing the scissoring technique we see in Sanseiru to do so.

The scissoring or arm-folding technique requires that the defender turn or pivot—"hidden" or at least not shown in the performance of the kata—pushing out and down against the opponent's arm with his or her outside arm and pulling in against the same arm with the defender's inside arm. This pushing out with the left arm and pull-ing in with the right arm—or vice versa—is sometimes shown when we begin Suparinpei (or Sanseiru), stepping into a right-foot-forward Basic Stance while bringing both arms up into the double-arm kamae posture. However, we might also use the first step into the double-arm kamae posture merely as an indication of the distance or that one has assumed a grappling posture similar to one's opponent. The scissoring or arm-folding techniques would not begin then until the step into the left-foot-forward posture. In any case, I would argue that the *rhythm* we usually see employed in this series of three steps and accompanying "punches" is what we might use to *teach* these movements but that the *application* (or bunkai) for these movements might actually employ a different kind of rhythm—one where the step into the left-foot-forward Basic Stance, for example, accompanies the left arm being brought back into the double-arm kamae. Similarly, after the right "punch," the right foot would step forward into a right-foot-forward Basic Stance as the right arm is brought back into the double-arm kamae. In other words, the movements of the arms and legs would be coordinated, the retraction of the "punching" arm accompanying the step forward. In the first step into a right-foot-forward Basic Stance to begin the kata, we would be using the scissoring or arm-folding technique against the opponent's right arm, turning to his outside or toward the east if we begin facing north. In the second step into a left-foot-forward Basic Stance, we would be using the scissoring or arm-folding technique against the opponent's left arm. When we *teach* kata, of course, we break all of the movements down into smaller, separate fragments—teaching one movement at a time—in order to make learning a kata easier. And for the most part, we retain this sort of staccato or punctuated movement whether we have just learned the kata or whether we've been practicing the movements for years.

The Double-Arm Spreading Technique

See figures 3.16–17.

In the next technique of Suparinpei kata, both hands are brought into the center, at a position just in front of the sternum, and then pushed out to the sides at shoulder level. The body sinks slightly as the arms are brought in and rises as the arms are thrust out.

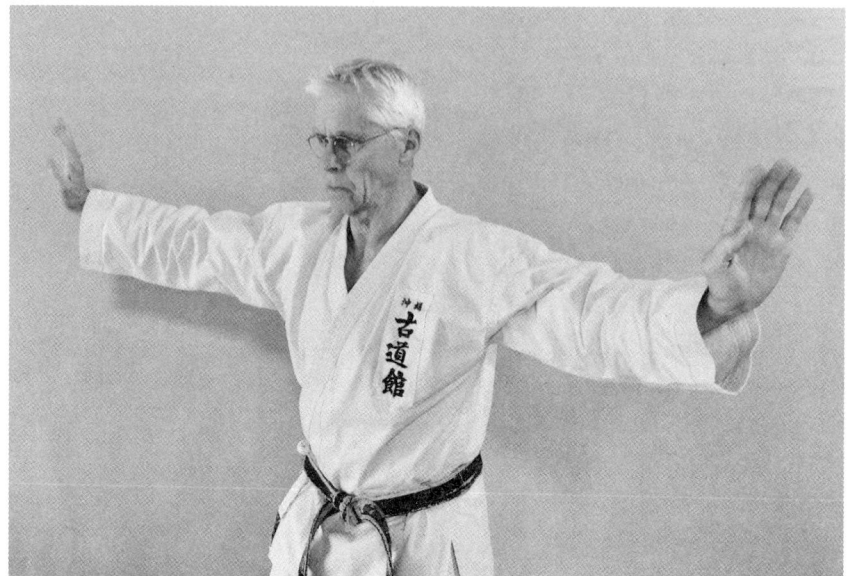

FIGURE 2.6 Both arms are used to spread the arms of the attacker.

This technique, again, should be understood in the context established by the opening double-arm kamae posture; that is, this technique is a response to a grapple or clinch. In the conventional interpretation of this technique, the opponent's arms are outside of the defender's arms or pushing in toward the center. The defender brings both hands inside the attacker's arms and, pushing out with both hands, separates the attacker's arms. From this position, inside the opponent's arms, the defender is in a much more advantageous position to counterattack. This arm-spreading technique may also be adapted to a scenario where the opponent's arms are on the outside of the defender's arms. In applying the technique, the defender pivots as the arms are brought in. As the arms push out, the defender's left hand holds or pushes against the opponent's left arm as the defender's right hand goes out to attack and grab the opponent's head (see fig. 2.8). From this position, the technique might continue with the rest of the mawashi uke and nukite/shuto sequence.

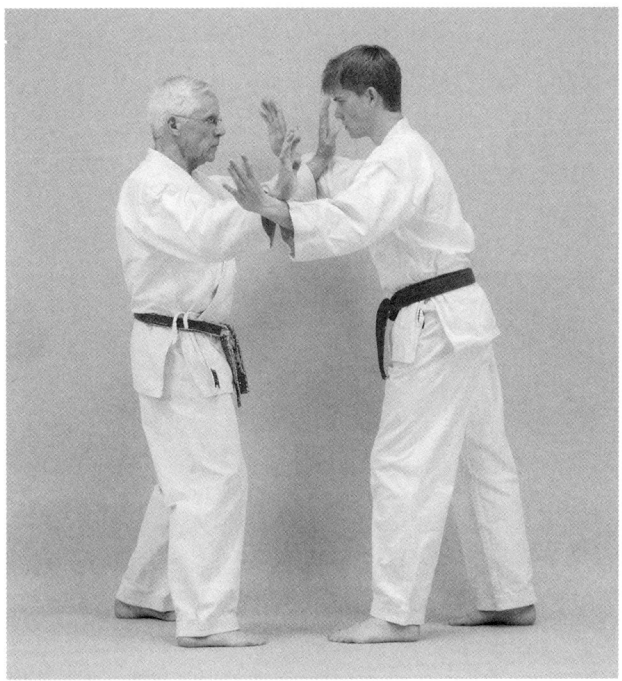

FIGURE 2.7 When the opponent attacks with both arms—whether it is pushing, grabbing the lapels, or attempting to choke the defender—both arms are brought in and then thrust out to spread the attacker's arms.

This technique is shown as a single, double-arm technique. If the conventional interpretation is correct, there is no sequence or follow-up to this technique as we would see in most of the other classical kata. But Suparinpei is somewhat unique in that the first half of the kata shows a number of disconnected techniques, rather than the more standard string of techniques we see in the bunkai sequences in the second half of the kata. This disconnectedness has prompted many to see this spreading arms technique as a single-arm technique in application, where the defender blocks and grabs the attacker's arm and then, turning sideways to the opponent, attacks the opponent with the open palm of the other hand.

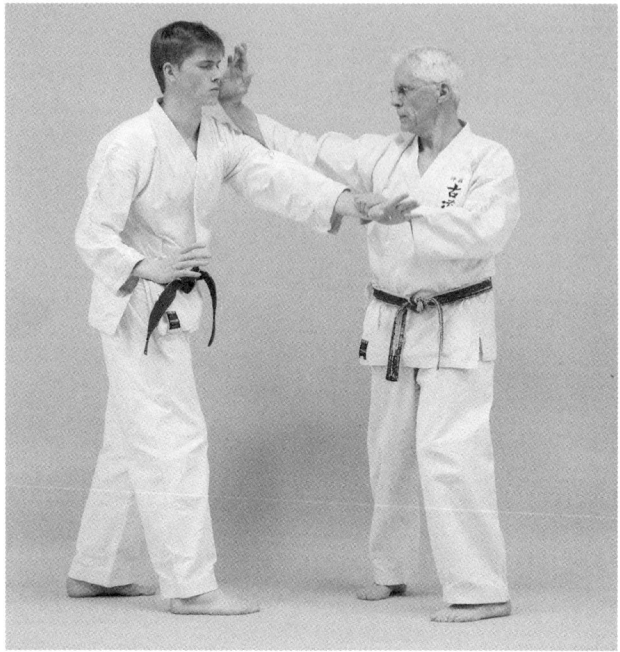

FIGURE 2.8 If we were to use the double-arm spreading technique as a single-hand grab and palm strike, it might look something like this.

This sort of interpretation, I believe, is a natural outgrowth of our expectations. We expect karate to be about hitting and kicking—an expectation borne out by any number of training models—and so we tend to look for explanations that fit our expectations. Whether the opponent is attacking with the conventional karate punch, lunging in with *zenkutsu dachi* (Front Stance), or grabbing the throat, we tend to look for an interpretation that will satisfy our own expectations of a karate-like counterattack—something we have trained. So our interpretation generally incorporates our own percussive attack.

We assume, therefore, that the attacker is punching, using the conventional karate straight punch, even if we have to turn sideways, compromising the position actually shown in kata, and turn one open hand into a grab of the opponent's punching arm and the other into a palm strike. It is more important, however, to see how this technique relates to what we see as one of the overall themes of the kata—how to deal with the opponent in a close-in or grappling situation. It would seem to be an almost reflexive action to bring both hands inside the attacker's arms and push out in order to deal with an opponent who has grabbed or attacked with both arms. However, the conventional application for this technique is not necessarily the best application.

The other, and it would seem more likely, application for this double-arm spreading technique has to do with its connection to the previous scissoring technique that we see in the opening set of three slow "punches." The techniques we see demonstrated in the first half of the kata—and that would include this double-arm spreading technique—seem to be a fragmented collection of individual techniques only because the structure, or how they are connected, isn't immediately apparent, and certainly not as straightforward as the three sequences we see in the second half of the kata, with their entry techniques, controlling or bridging techniques, and finishing techniques. However, if we use the scissoring technique we see illustrated with the three "punches" in the opening series of the kata (see fig. 2.5), then the opponent's head is brought in and down as the double-arm folding technique is applied.

After the last slow "punch" with the left hand, the arm is pulled back, bringing the hands together in front of the chest. With the scissoring technique of the double-arm kamae, the opponent's arm is folded and the head is brought in and down so that the left "punch" is thrust out alongside the opponent's head (see fig. 2.9). When it is retracted, the defender's head is brought in. With one hand on the back of the attacker's head and one hand on the chin (see fig. 2.10)—this is illustrated by the opening of the hands after the last "punch"—the arms are then pushed out to the sides, twisting the opponent's head, an application that is more in keeping with what we see in the rest of the kata.

Sanseiru and Seisan also begin from the double-arm kamae posture followed by three "punches." In all three of these kata, I would suggest, the first two "punches" show a scissoring or arm-folding technique, first against the opponent's left arm and then against the opponent's right arm.

The third "punch" in each kata is used to bring the opponent's head back into a position that allows the defender to control or twist the head, or, in the case of Sanseiru, to grab the opponent's head with the open right hand technique and pull the opponent down. None of these techniques are punches, and only the first two of each sequence function similarly. The third "punch" in each case acts as a linking or bridging technique between the arm-folding or scissoring entry technique and the head-twisting finishing techniques of the rest of the sequence.

In this case, it is difficult to know which application may have been the application the individual or individuals who created this kata originally intended, or which application seems the more likely given the structure of the kata. In sequences this short, it is hard to say what the structure or apparent lack of structure is trying to convey. It is tempting to look at the double-arm spreading technique as a separate technique, not a part of any sequence, intended to offer another method of dealing with a clinch

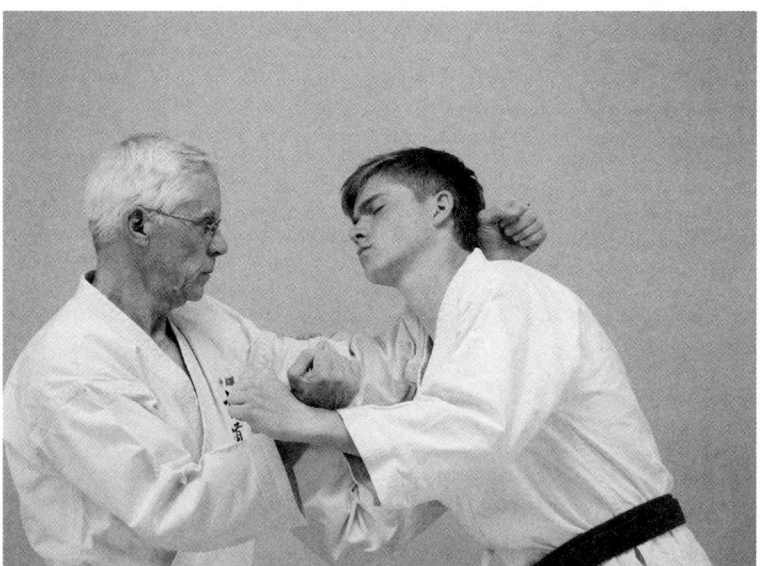

FIGURE 2.9 Because of the use of the scissor-like arm-folding technique, what appears to be a middle-level punch *(chudan tsuki)* is positioned to the side of the attacker's head.

scenario—in this case, showing one method of dealing with an opponent who has grabbed the defender or who has both arms on the outside of the defender's arms. The other entry techniques that we see in both the first half and the second half of the kata show methods of dealing with other grappling-like scenarios—that is, with one arm on the inside and one arm on the outside, or with both arms outside the attacker's arms.

One of the problems, however, is that if the opponent is strong and actually grabbing the defender, then this double-arm spreading technique requires a good deal of strength to break the opponent's grasp. The second problem is that the other techniques of the kata—even the seemingly fragmented section of the first half that begins with the mawashi uke techniques and ends with the shiko dachi angle techniques—are all part of application sequences, showing entry, bridging, and finishing techniques. (This is covered later in the text.) And though it is certainly possible, it seems less likely that there are one or two techniques stuck here at the

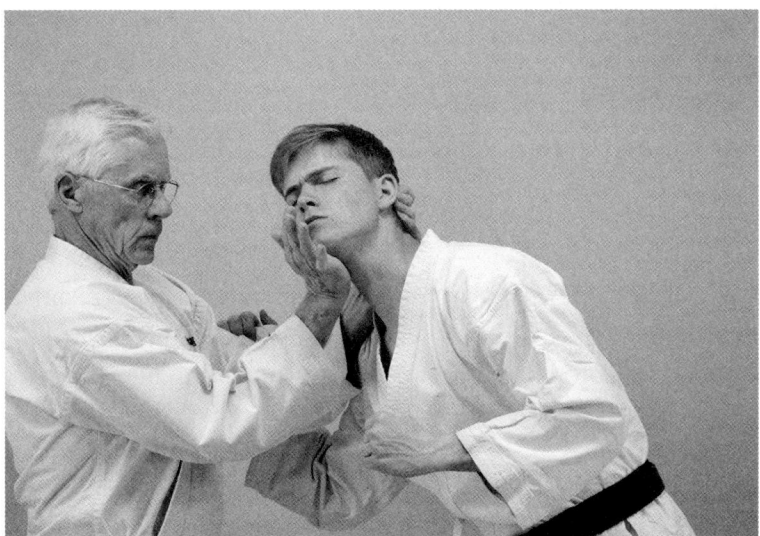

FIGURE 2.10 In the performance of the kata, we bring both arms in toward the chest prior to the double-arm spreading technique. In application, the last "punch" is used to bring the opponent's head in after the last scissoring or folding technique of the double-arm kamae.

beginning of the kata that are shown as individual techniques, taken out of context, as it were.

A further argument one might make is that the third "punch" in each of the related kata—that is, Sanseiru and Seisan—is used to bring the opponent's head in after the use of the scissoring or arm-folding technique and before a head-twisting technique. In other words, if we look at the opening techniques of these kata in this way, then they are not showing *three* punches but a right scissoring technique, a left scissoring technique, and then a scissoring technique used with the retraction of the left arm into an open-hand head grab and neck-twisting technique.

I think it is far more likely, and perhaps just structurally more satisfying, to say that there are three entry techniques illustrated in the kata—the beginning double-arm kamae that acts as a scissoring or folding technique, the mawashi uke in Basic Stance, and the semicircular dropping and rising arm blocks that begin each of the sequences of the second half—with, of course, their accompanying finishing head-twisting techniques, like the double-arm spreading technique here.

The Double *Mawashi Uke* and Left *Nukite/ Shuto* Technique

See figures 3.18–25.

The next series of techniques—the right and left mawashi uke and nukite/shuto—may be one of the most fundamental and important techniques in Suparinpei. (It is difficult to say whether this open hand position, where the left hand is brought in, palm up, after the mawashi uke and right hand grab, is a nukite or shuto attack, or whether it is simply an open hand that comes in to control the opponent's chin.) It may also be one of the most misunderstood, however useful. In fact, the mawashi uke seems so ubiquitous at times, and so cryptic, if you will, that it has prompted all manner of speculation about how it may be used. The circular movements of the arms have been dissected until it seems as though it's a technique with almost infinite possibilities, as if all you might need in any situation

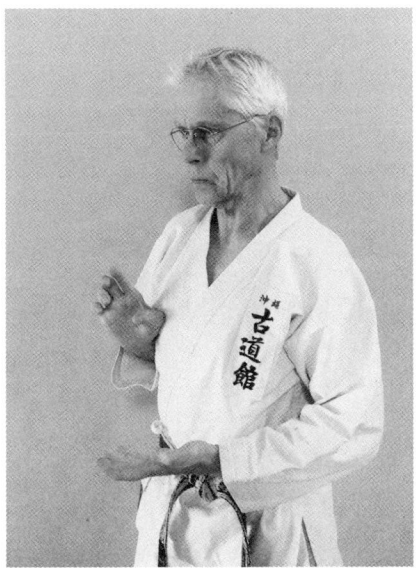

FIGURE 2.11 The head grab and
nukite position at the end of the
mawashi uke.

dealing with an attacker is a thorough understanding of the mawashi uke
(think: "wax on; wax off").

This creative maelstrom of interpretations swirling around the mawashi
uke that one can find in numerous print publications and countless videos,
however, is fed largely by the notion that a kata is no more than a jumble
of individual techniques. If we take a technique out of context—out of the
sequence of moves in the kata—then there is no way to determine how it
was meant to function. And if we don't understand the *structure* of a kata,
how and why the techniques are put together, then it is almost impossible
to see it in any other way. To add to this difficulty, there is not one uniform
structure or set of rules that can be applied to all of the koryu (classical)
kata within a particular system. There are similarities between the patterns of different kata, but again there don't seem to be universal rules we
can use to decipher kata. However, simply because the structures of the
various classical kata differ, it doesn't mean there *isn't* a structure. Simply

because there isn't a single key that will unlock each door in a house doesn't mean that we can't open all of the doors if we find the keys. Or, at the very least, just because there doesn't seem to be a single key we can use to unlock the structure or pattern of all of the Goju classical subjects, it doesn't mean we can't find the best explanation for the techniques of kata.

The structure may be difficult to see, but that doesn't mean we should abandon the task in favor of what, at present, seems to be a more widely held opinion, but to my thinking much less defendable, that the techniques of kata can mean anything you want them to mean. If this were indeed the case, it would be like taking a word that we were unfamiliar with and trying to define it without any of the contextual clues we would have if we were to see it in a sentence or see that sentence in a larger paragraph. Without context the meaning is left open to wildly speculative interpretation, the imagination given free bent, as anyone who has played the dictionary game knows. But, as I will try to point out, there are what we might call contextual clues.

The mawashi uke we see at the beginning of Suparinpei kata is done in Basic Stance—an important distinction. This only occurs in two other kata in the Goju canon: Sanchin and Tensho. Each of these kata begins from the double-arm kamae posture, significant because it establishes the range or the posture with which one is confronting the attacker, and one that assumes the opponent has taken up a similar position. It might also be assumed, therefore, that the mawashi technique here is dealing with the opponent's arms in the middle frame—that is, the defender is using the mawashi uke against an opponent's push or another kind of grappling scenario where the opponent is attacking with both hands rather than the typical karate punch or chudan tsuki directed at the defender's mid-section.

This is not to say that the mawashi uke is altogether ineffective against a straight chudan punch, only that this kind of attack—one that we often see in paired ippon kumite or *yakusoku kumite* drills in the dojo—is not very realistic. We often use it in the dojo because it is a safer way to practice, particularly with junior students. The mawashi uke we see here, in Basic Stance, covering the middle frame or middle level, is used to counter the pushing or pulling attack of an opponent using both arms.

To see this more clearly, we can position ourselves in front of a training partner in a right-foot-forward Basic Stance with both arms held up in front of the body—the same position we adopt at the beginning of Suparinpei kata. (Suparinpei is the last of the Kaishu or "open-hand" kata in the Goju canon. Just like the old stories that Sanchin was once upon a time an open-hand kata—that Miyagi Chojun sensei closed the hands in his version of Sanchin—Suparinpei, I believe, probably began with an open-hand kamae, perhaps similar to Shisochin kata or the opening position we see in many White Crane kung fu forms, or for that matter, in the Uechi-ryu version of Sanchin kata.) If we use a grappling-like posture, we might have both of our arms outside our partner's arms, or we might have one arm outside and one arm inside. The position we are starting from is somewhat akin to a free-form pushing-hands drill one might encounter in any Chinese-based martial art.

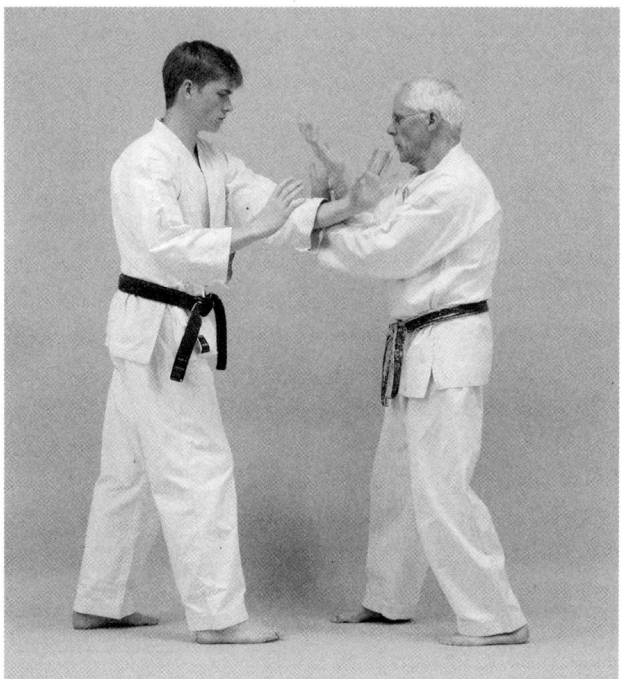

FIGURE 2.12 The right arm pushes in on the attacker's left arm.

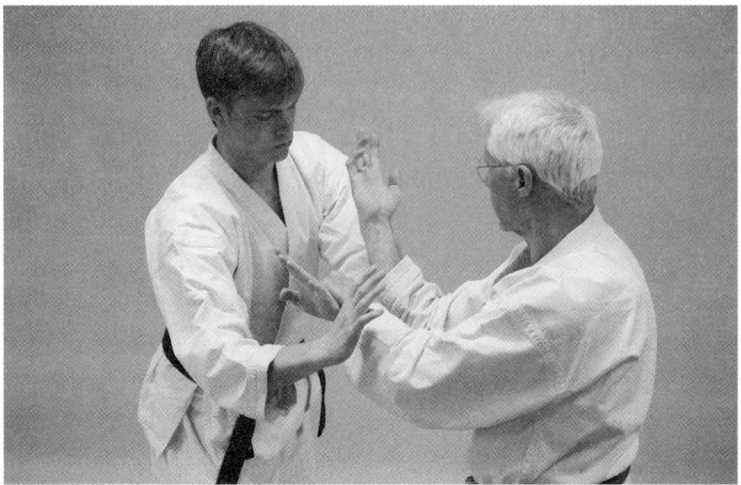

FIGURE 2.13 The left hand comes around and under to grab the attacker's left wrist, twisting it to bring the head down. Though the full twisting motion is not shown here, this would be the position of the left hand we see in the solo kata performance of this technique, with the palm forward and the fingers pointing down.

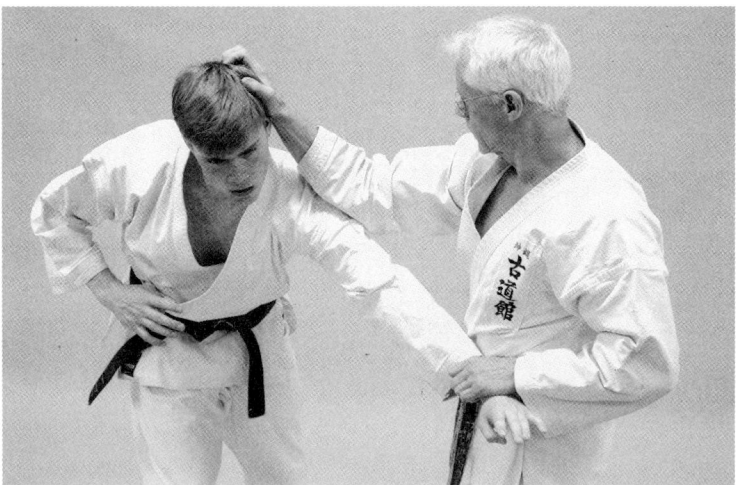

FIGURE 2.14 The right hand comes up to grab the opponent's head or hair. This is the position of the right hand that we see in the solo kata performance of the mawashi, with the palm forward and the fingers pointing up.

So, for example, with both parties in a right-foot-forward Basic Stance, and the left arm on the inside and the right arm on the outside (or, in fact, both of the defender's arms on the outside), imagine the attacker pushing in, toward the defender's center, with his left arm, in order to unbalance the defender. (In practicing any of the techniques based on the mawashi uke in two-person or partner drills, it is important to remember that the opponent is pushing in or attacking. The mawashi uke is not nearly as effective if both sides are merely standing still in a kind of stasis.) The defender uses the first mawashi uke we see in the opening of Suparinpei kata to fold or push the attacker's left arm in toward the center, while the defender's left arm comes underneath the attacker's left arm, grabbing it at the wrist (see fig. 2.13).

Then twisting the attacker's arm, the defender's right hand comes up to grab the attacker's hair or head (see fig. 2.14), pulling in as the left open hand or nukite/shuto comes in to attack the neck or control the chin (see fig. 2.15). (The position of the defender's right and left hands, prior to the nukite/shuto, looks the same as the position of the hands in the classical mawashi uke posture from kata; that is, with the twisting of the opponent's left arm, the defender's left hand is more or less palm-forward with the fingers pointing down, while the defender's right palm, with the fingers pointing up, is facing forward prior to being brought up to grab the attacker's head.) As the kata suggests, of course, the mawashi uke is facilitated by a step or turn in the direction of the technique or stepping off line—that is, turning in a counterclockwise direction as the right mawashi uke is applied against the attacker's left arm. (Notice that when one applies the right-side mawashi uke, pushing in with the right arm, with the counterclockwise turn, the left foot is forward, as it is in kata. The left nukite/shuto is applied as one steps forward with the right foot.)

This "nukite/shuto" is the same technique we see at the beginning of Seiunchin kata, though in that sequence it is executed after an arm bar, which itself is a response to a cross-hand wrist grab (see fig. 1.14). It may be interesting to note that this is the opposite-side or left-hand-to-left-hand wrist grab that necessitates the initial response or first technique of Seiunchin kata. In other words, if the attacker were using this initial mawashi uke technique with its left-hand grab against the defender, then the first technique in Seiunchin kata might be used as an effective counter. In fact, the techniques we see in Saifa and Seiunchin serve as counterattacks to two of the initial entry techniques, both of which employ wrist grabs, of Suparinpei kata. Seiunchin techniques serve as counters to the cross-hand wrist grabs we see in the series of mawashi uke and nukite/shuto techniques at the beginning of the kata. Saifa techniques serve as counters to the same-side wrist grabs we see in the entry techniques that begin each of the sequences of the second half of the kata.

However, in the case of Seiunchin, this head grab and nukite/shuto is not used as a finishing technique but merely a controlling technique that allows us to move into the elbow technique to the back of the opponent's neck and, most probably, using the final technique of the kata—the *yama uke* (mountain block) and *hiza geri* or knee kick—as the finishing technique. Because of the similarity between the nukite at the beginning of Seiunchin and the

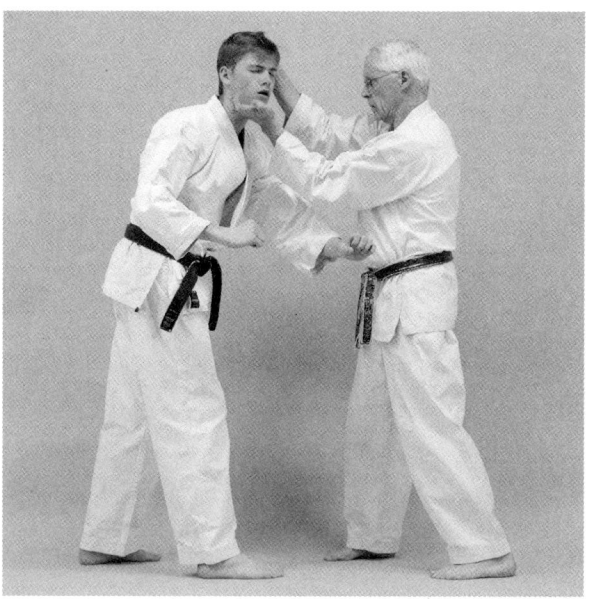

FIGURE 2.15 After the mawashi uke, the right hand pulls the opponent's head in as the left "nukite/shuto" comes in to attack and control the chin.

nukite/shuto here at the beginning of Suparinpei, I would argue that this is not meant to be a finishing technique in Suparinpei either, that this mawashi uke and nukite/shuto merely shows the initial receiving technique and the bridging or controlling technique. The finishing techniques are the series of three techniques—one shown three times and the other two shown four times each—that follow the series of double mawashi uke techniques.

But if that is the case, why structure the kata this way? Why not show a full sequence with a single mawashi uke followed by a mawashi head-twisting technique in Cat Stance, then another single mawashi uke followed by a head-twisting double punch, and then another single mawashi uke followed by another head-twisting technique performed in shiko dachi to the corner? Why not make the sequences easier to "see" and understand? Were the creators of these kata—whoever put together these sequences of individual techniques—trying to hide the actual applications?

The answer, I suspect, is that there *is* no particular reason; either way would be fine. Showing complete sequences may be clearer—as we see in most of the sequences of Seipai kata, for instance—but if the aim is to show the versatility of the mawashi uke as a receiving or entry technique, then the traditional structure that we see in Suparinpei, with its four repetitions of the right and left mawashi uke techniques, is sufficient, provided the student understands the structure. The problem for any of us trying to understand the structure, however, is that no other classical subjects use repetitions of four unless they are repeating techniques that at least in application should be paired, as we see in the "elbow" techniques of Seiunchin kata or the open-palm techniques of Shisochin. In the first of these cases, Seiunchin, the application of the "elbow" techniques requires that two of the four techniques be used together. This is also the case with the four open-palm techniques in the middle section of Shisochin.

In the case of Shisochin kata, the repetition of the four angular forearm techniques may be used to show variations in how they are applied. These variations may be one explanation for subtle differences in how various schools perform the same kata. The bunkai remains largely the same, but the performance of the kata differs. (This is also true of many of the differences we see in the performance of Sanseiru kata as well.)

I suspect, however, that the angular forearm techniques of Shisochin are actually closer to what we see in Suparinpei—that is, they are not meant to be applied in combination but simply to show both the right and left side applications. The first of these angular forearm techniques, stepping out to the northeast, is used to unbalance and bring the opponent's head down after the initial scissoring technique against the opponent's left arm, and then, pivoting, attack the head using the right forearm (see fig. A.8 and figs. 2.16–17). The second of these angular forearm techniques, stepping out to the northwest, is used to unbalance and bring the opponent's head down after the initial scissoring technique against the opponent's right arm, and then, pivoting, attack the head using the left forearm.

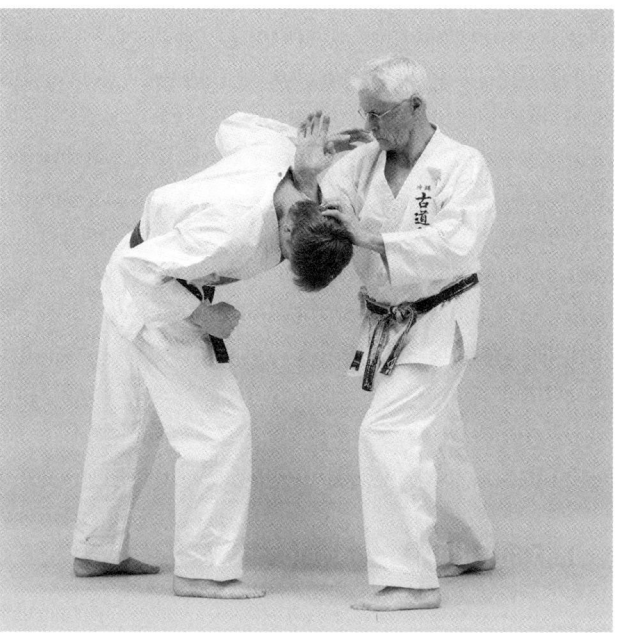

FIGURE 2.16 This attack to the opponent's neck, from the first sequence of Shisochin kata, is shown first using the right forearm and then using the left forearm in order to show both sides.

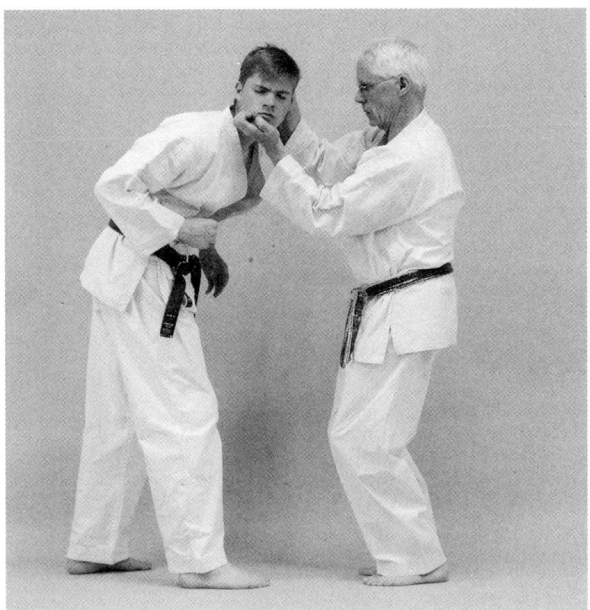

FIGURE 2.17 In application, this head-twisting technique
would follow the attack with the right forearm in Shisochin. The hand that is used to attack the neck is used to
control the head, while the hand that is grabbing the hair
is brought up into the opponent's chin, twisting the head.
The first kata sequence only shows the head-twisting
finish of the left forearm attack, while the same sequence
in the second half of the kata shows the finish of the right
forearm attack.

This separation of techniques is closer to what we see with the mawashi
uke techniques of Suparinpei. Here, the paired mawashi uke techniques
are meant to be taken apart. The kata is showing first a right mawashi uke
and then, after stepping forward, a left mawashi uke. This is markedly
different from what we generally see in the other classical subjects.

Since this is the first technique, or more properly first series, that is
repeated four times, it would be fair to ask, why? One can only guess. Perhaps they are repeated four times because there are four techniques in this

first half of the kata, before the first complete bunkai sequence. Or perhaps it is to emphasize the four cardinal and four ordinal directions, as if to remind us of the admonition in the Happo: "The eyes see in four directions; the ears hear in eight directions." Or perhaps it's simply aesthetic.

Another difference is that the right-hand grab and left nukite attack to the neck or chin of the opponent is, I believe, meant to be attached to the first mawashi uke in each series. This also differs from what we see in most of the other kata, where the finishing technique, usually shown only once, is tacked onto the end of the second sequence when we have a repetition of techniques or a sequence that is shown on both sides. At the end of Seiunchin, for example, the finishing technique—the left-hand grab and forearm strike followed by the yama uke and hiza geri—is shown only after the second series of "elbow" techniques. At the end of Saifa, the finishing technique—the final mawashi-*like* head twist and knee kick (the last position of the kata)—is again shown only once, after the second series that began with the left-foot sweep and hammer fist. In Seiunchin kata the finishing technique of the opening series is shown only once, but the head grab and nukite attack is shown on both the right and left sides, since the opening series is done three times. In Suparinpei the left-hand head grab and right nukite—what would follow the second or left-side mawashi uke—is not shown. The right-hand head grab and left nukite attack in the first series of Seiunchin, however, looks the same in application as it does here in Suparinpei, except in Seiunchin it is done in shiko dachi.

All of this may seem like an overly cerebral dissection of kata. But when we compare similar techniques in different classical subjects, it helps in our understanding of kata and reinforces our interpretations of the applications.

One last note should probably be mentioned here regarding the head grab and nukite we see as part of this mawashi uke series in Suparinpei, particularly as it relates to Seiunchin. When we see this technique performed in either kata, the right hand is rotated up from the down position, pausing with the elbow down and the right open palm facing up. This appears to be a distinct move because of the timing or rhythm used in its execution, which is probably due to the piecemeal manner we generally adopt to teach kata.

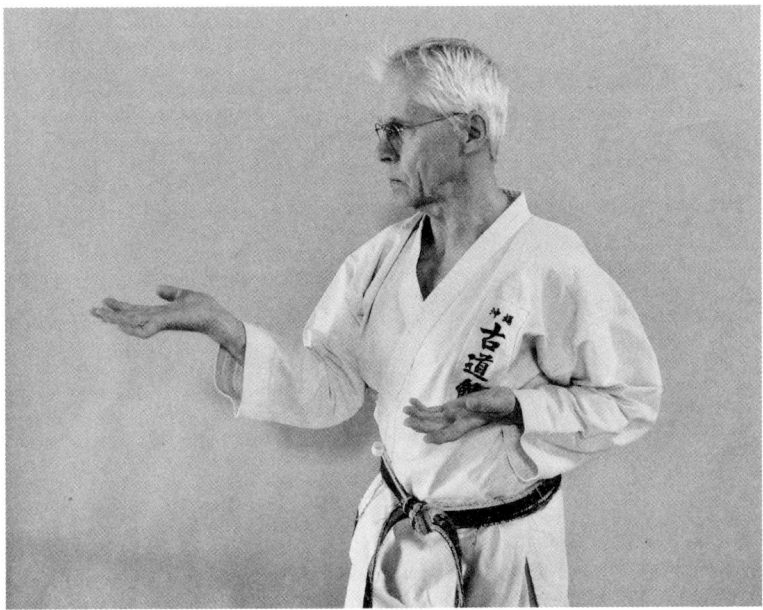

FIGURE 2.18 This palm-up technique from the mawashi uke sequence in Suparinpei is meant to ensure that the elbow is kept down in the execution of the head grab, but it is not meant to be a separate technique.

Because of these pauses, however, students generally look for a separate application for each of these movements. Most often, the interpretation is that the right arm is brought up to block another of the opponent's punches. Then the right hand is rotated so that the open hand faces forward or down, grabbing the opponent's arm. The right hand is then pulled in as the left open hand, palm up, is thrust out to attack the opponent's ribs. I would suggest, however, though it may be a bit difficult to describe, that in the case of Seiunchin kata, the right arm is rotated up with the elbow down, as the left hand twists the opponent's arm, so that the defender can use his or her right forearm to keep pressure against the opponent's elbow—the effect of this technique, however subtle it may appear, is to maintain control of the opponent and prevent against the attacker initiating an attack with the left elbow. Though less obvious, this may also be the case with Suparinpei.

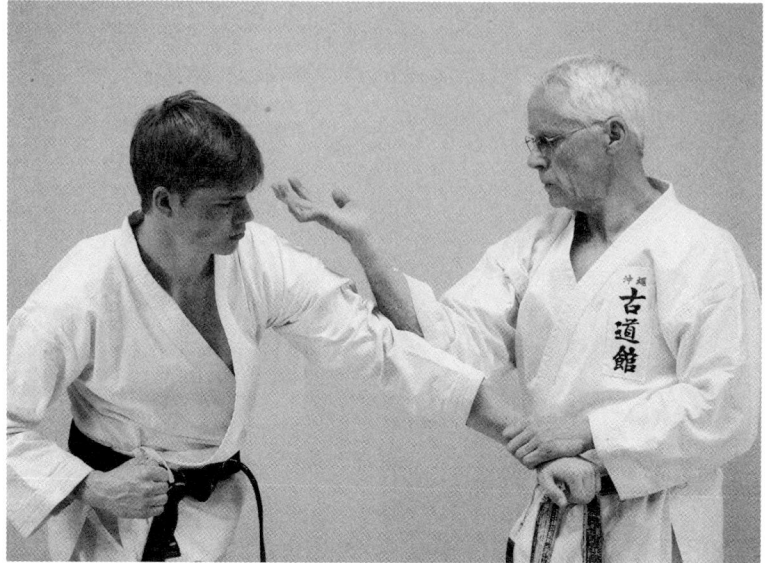

FIGURE 2.19 In this close-up of the mawashi application, we can see how the forearm is used to control the opponent's arm prior to the right-hand head grab and left nukite.

In any event, the palm-up position should not be treated as a separate technique, nor should there be a distinct pause in its execution in solo kata. The hand should be brought up and rotated in a single fluid movement in order to best effect the right-hand grab of the opponent's head. Anything else is not only too slow but unrealistic.

The *Mawashi* in Cat Stance

See figures 3.26–28.

I wrote a good deal about the mawashi techniques in my first book,[8] so I will just briefly explain that I am convinced from years of study, and a good deal of trial and error, that there are really two kinds of mawashi techniques in the Goju classical kata: the mawashi uke technique, which is executed in Basic Stance, and the mawashi-like technique, which is executed in Cat Stance *(neko ashi dachi)*. We find both techniques in Suparinpei

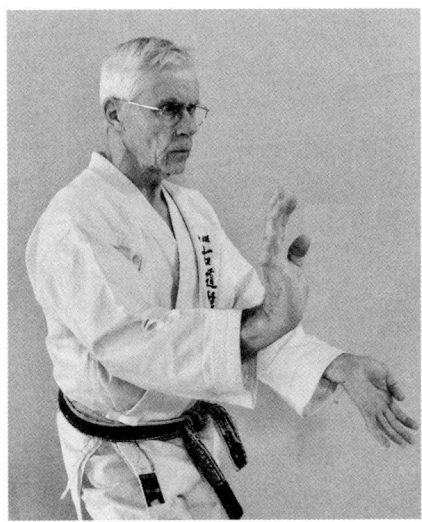

FIGURE 2.20 The end position of the hands in the mawashi-like technique and the mawashi uke is the same. The only difference is the stance.

kata. The problem, I believe, in understanding how these techniques are meant to be applied is that the circular arm movements are often done the same when they were never intended to be exactly the same.

Simply put, the mawashi in Basic Stance is a receiving or "blocking" technique, while the mawashi in Cat Stance is a finishing technique—the Cat Stance in Goju-ryu generally signifying the use of a kick or an attack with the front knee. The Cat Stance mawashi always occurs at the *end* of an application sequence, using the knee to attack what is being held in the hands. The logical answer is that the hands have grasped the opponent's head. Since the hands rotate in the mawashi technique, the suggestion is that the head or neck is twisted. And the front knee would most likely be brought up not at the completion of the mawashi technique but partway through its execution.

The two terms most often used for these mawashi techniques—*mawashi uke* and *tora guchi*—have long been in use, but there has been little agreement on the difference between them, some using them interchangeably. I would suggest that *tora guchi* is probably a more appropriate term to use when the mawashi technique is used to seize and hold the opponent like the jaws of a tiger. Fittingly, this is usually signaled by the use of the Cat Stance—as we see it, for example, at the end of Saifa kata or in the middle of Kururunfa kata. The mawashi uke technique, on the other hand, is used as an initial receiving technique, and it is executed in Basic Stance.

The problem in using even this relatively easy method of distinguishing between these two terms, however, is illustrated in the series of paired mawashi uke techniques at the beginning of Suparinpei. The mawashi uke is used at the start of the encounter to neutralize the opponent's push (see fig. 2.12), for example, but the defender's left hand is then used to seize

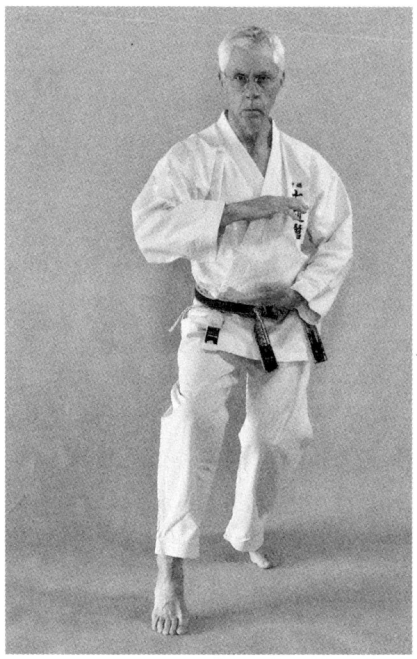

FIGURE 2.21 The beginning of the mawashi from the middle of Kururunfa kata. Both hands are holding the opponent's head prior to twisting in a clockwise direction and attacking with the knee.

the opponent's left wrist (fig. 2.13) while the defender's right hand is used to seize the opponent's head (fig. 2.14). In this case, the blocking or receiving action occurs at the beginning of the technique while the seizing and attacking action occurs at the end of the technique. This has led some to suggest that the technique itself should be referred to as a mawashi uke/tora guchi—that it is, in fact, both, at least in Suparinpei, and that the use of the single term *mawashi uke* was merely a shorthand reference, or whichever term one uses depends on which part of the technique one is describing.

However, all of this may seem needlessly complicated (even perhaps a little pedantic), and since there is really no general agreement on when to use one term and when to use the other, I will refer to one as the mawashi uke or mawashi in Basic Stance and the other as the mawashi-*like* technique or the mawashi in Cat Stance.

One should note, however, that the distinction is not just in which stance is used, though this is quite important in deciphering applications. The arm movements, I would argue, are also a bit different. Conventionally, the arm movements, at least in the performance of Suparinpei kata, are executed in the same manner for either mawashi technique (see fig. 2.22). For example, in a left-foot-forward Cat Stance—as we see in the second of three Cat Stance mawashi techniques at this point in Suparinpei kata—the right forearm is raised vertically as the left hand is brought down, under the right elbow. Then the left hand circles toward the left hip while the right hand is pulled back and rotated. At the completion of the circular arm movements, with the palms facing forward, the left hand pointing down and the right hand pointing up, the hands push forward (see fig. 2.20). This is essentially the same way that the mawashi uke technique in Basic Stance is usually performed in kata. Yet they function quite differently.

The forward pushing motion at the end of the mawashi, done slowly and often with dynamic tension, has led some to assume that the mawashi in Cat Stance is a pushing technique. One of the problems with this, however, is that the use of a Cat Stance to push an opponent doesn't really make sense—it's not a strong stance, nor is it very stable. (It also doesn't seem to fit the general tenor of the Goju classical subjects, where the lethal nature of the finishing techniques is intended to end an encounter.) Those that make this argument tend to look for rationalizations that don't seem to help all that much either—that the Cat Stance is employed in order to use a kick to facilitate the push, or that the original stance was probably a Front Stance but that early practitioners hid the real technique by disguising it as a Cat Stance. In any event, why would one push the attacker away simply to begin the encounter all over again?

For me, these sorts of explanations so often evoke Ockham's razor. It's much easier to explain the Cat Stance and apparent "push" with the hands if we can imagine the defender using this finishing mawashi-like technique to grasp the opponent by the head—as the tiger would seize its prey in its jaws. The head or neck is twisted and pushed out, away from the body, in order to bring the knee up. This is the finish to most of the mawashi-like techniques in the Goju classical kata. (The mawashi-like technique in Cat Stance is done in kata at the chudan level because the previous entry technique has brought the opponent's head down to this level.)

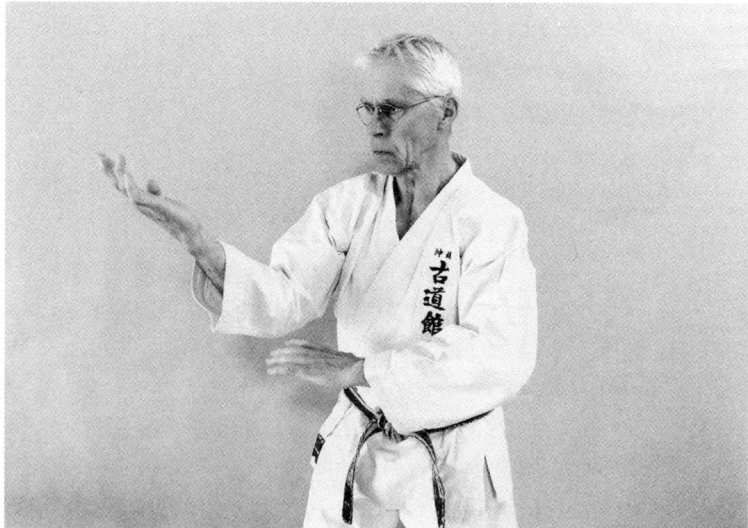

FIGURE 2.22 The conventional starting position of the arms is usually the same whether it is showing the mawashi uke in Basic Stance or the mawashi in Cat Stance.

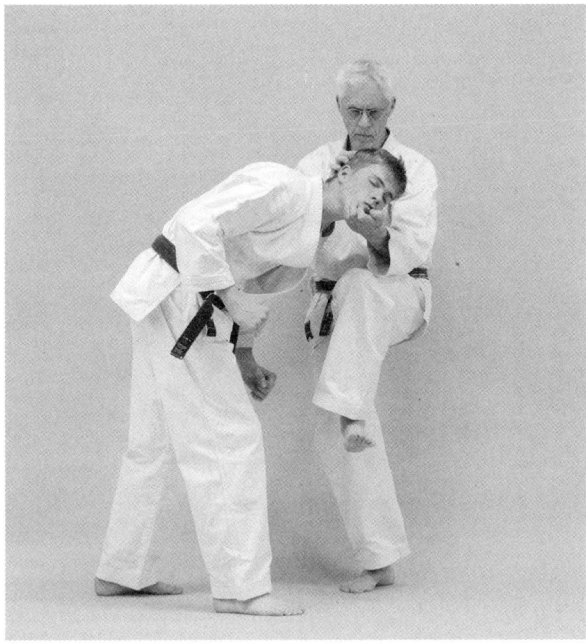

FIGURE 2.23 The mawashi technique in neko ashi dachi is used to seize the opponent's head and attack with the front knee.

The simple mawashi-like technique that we see here, for example, and at the end of Saifa or in the middle of Kururunfa kata, is different from the opening mawashi uke because in this case the defender is already grasping the opponent's head—one hand holding the chin while the other hand is holding the head or grabbing the hair, arriving at this position, of course, by first employing the mawashi uke and nukite/shuto entry technique. From this position, it is simply a matter of rotating the hands and arms into the final mawashi position, which is the same in both mawashi techniques, and attacking with the knee kick or hiza geri. The hands move in a clockwise circle (in the first of these techniques, and counterclockwise in the second), as if they are moving around the surface of a ball. This is the technique, I would argue, that is used here, in Suparinpei, after the initial mawashi uke in Basic Stance.

In some respects, of course, it is an oversimplification to reduce the mawashi techniques we encounter in the classical kata of Goju-ryu to one or the other of these two methods of execution. Many of the finishing techniques begin from this position with one hand controlling the head while the other hand is pulling or pushing on the opponent's chin. The two hands work in opposition and, depending on the position of the opponent, the finishing techniques are executed in a variety of planes of motion. Essentially, they all function the same way—twisting the head or breaking the attacker's neck or simply throwing the attacker to the ground (depending on how much force is applied to the twisting motion)—but they may appear to be different.

Admittedly, there is some argument to execute the head-twisting mawashi in Cat Stance in almost the same manner as the conventional mawashi uke described above, though here again there are subtle differences. In this case, beginning from the same initial entry technique of this sequence, the right-side mawashi uke with right-hand head grab and left nukite/shuto technique (see fig. 2.15), the defender's right hand would push down on the opponent's head as the defender's left hand pushed up on the opponent's chin, twisting the head. This is the starting position of the conventional mawashi uke illustrated above (fig. 2.22).

From here, the left hand pulls back on the opponent's chin as the right hand rotates, pushing down toward the defender's right hip, twisting the opponent's head back in the other direction. This is another way of executing the mawashi in Cat Stance. It looks similar to the execution of the mawashi uke (receiving technique), but the arms in this case do not cross; that is, the right hand that is used to push down on the attacker's head does *not* pass under the defender's left elbow.

Interestingly, there is also a third way one might execute this mawashi technique in Cat Stance. In this case, we have to imagine the first of the three mawashi in Cat Stance of this series (facing west) coming off the opposite-side or left mawashi uke instead of the right mawashi uke. The technique would start from the end position of the left mawashi uke—that is, the left hand has been brought up to grab the head, and the right hand has been brought into the neck or chin of the opponent. This is the head grab and nukite/shuto that is *not* shown in kata. The suggestion is that each of the finishing techniques that follow the mawashi uke—the mawashi in Cat Stance, the double punch, and the angular shiko dachi series—comes off the left-side mawashi uke combination or the one not fully demonstrated in the kata. This is suggested primarily by the hair-grabbing technique that begins the shiko dachi angle sequence (see below).

As the defender shifts back into a right-foot-forward Cat Stance (or the first one shown in kata), the right hand pushes out and up on the opponent's chin as the left hand continues to hold the head. Then the head is twisted as both hands rotate into the final mawashi position with the left hand pointing up and the right hand pointing down, both palms forward—that is, the head is first twisted in one direction, and then twisted back in the opposite direction. In practice, this manner of executing the head-twisting mawashi in Cat Stance looks very much like the conventional mawashi uke, except once again the arms do *not* cross—the right hand does not pass under the defender's left elbow. And, like the earlier description of this mawashi in Cat Stance, the circle described by the rotating hands would be considerably smaller than what we usually see in the performance of this kata technique. After all, the hands are positioned on the opponent's head, so any exaggeratedly large arm motions would be unrealistic.

It should also be remembered that no matter which method one uses in executing the mawashi in Cat Stance, the head-twisting application of this technique often *requires a directional change or turn*—the use of the 90-degree or 180-degree directional changes one sees in kata. In other words, if the attacker is pushing in or attacking with his left arm, the defender would turn slightly to avoid the push, executing a right mawashi uke, grabbing the attacker's arm with the left hand and grabbing the head with the right hand. Then, pivoting, which would require a step, either 90 degrees or 180 degrees to the right or clockwise, the defender would twist and attack the opponent's head, using the front knee of the Cat Stance. Interestingly, this technique—using the second Cat Stance mawashi with the left mawashi uke—can be performed in a simpler fashion if one utilizes a counterclockwise 90-degree turn while executing the technique. In this case, the left hand, which is holding the opponent's head or hair, simply pulls down toward the left knee, as the right hand, which is on the opponent's chin, pushes out.

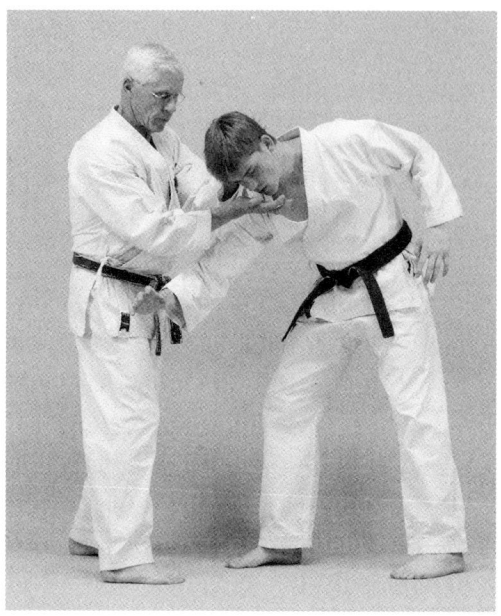

FIGURE 2.24 In the left mawashi uke technique, the left hand would grab the opponent's head as the right hand is brought in to attack the neck and control the chin.

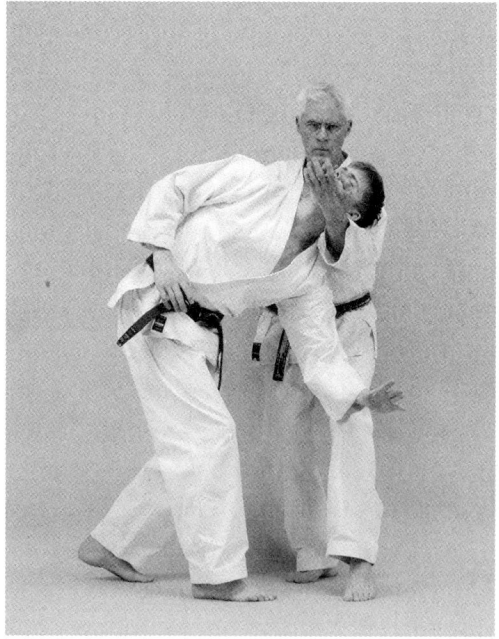

FIGURE 2.25 The first and third of the Cat Stance mawashi techniques probably begin from the right-hand head grab and left nukite/shuto (responding to a left attack from the opponent). The second of the Cat Stance mawashi techniques, shown here, probably begins from the left-hand head grab and right nukite/shuto by pushing in on the opponent's chin, remembering that in both cases the mawashi techniques are executed with a 90- or 180-degree turn.

The key to understanding the mawashi in Cat Stance is to understand the structure of the kata, and the structure of Suparinpei is somewhat peculiar, particularly when we compare it to most of the other classical subjects. There are some things that seem inconsistent. The mawashi in Cat Stance is one. Each of the other finishing techniques in the first half of the kata—the double punch and the angular shiko dachi technique (see below)—comes off the left-side mawashi uke or the second of the paired mawashi uke techniques. (It is worth noting that these techniques, coming as they do off the left-side mawashi uke, are consistent with what one would expect against a right-handed opponent attacking with his right hand or pushing in with the right arm. This would explain the emphasis the kata seems to show here.) The starting position for each of them—both are only shown on one side—would be the left-hand head grab and right-hand nukite/shuto. The problem is that this technique is *not* shown in the kata; the structure of the kata leaves out this crucial connection.

The mawashi in Cat Stance, however, may provide a sort of clue to solving this dilemma. Interestingly, this technique, shown three times, is the only one of these finishing techniques that is done on both the right and left sides, and consequently would be the only one that might be thought to illustrate the mawashi in Cat Stance off both the right-side mawashi uke, with its right-hand head grab and left nukite/shuto, and the left-side mawashi uke, with its left-hand head grab and right nukite/shuto.

It is certainly possible, however, depending on how exactly one executes the mawashi arm movements, that each of the Cat Stance mawashi techniques is meant to be applied from the left-side mawashi uke, the same as each of the two following finishing techniques. How one turns—that is, whether one turns 180 degrees in a counterclockwise direction or 90 degrees in a clockwise direction—may simply depend on the position of the opponent's body after the application of the initial mawashi uke. Structurally, this makes a lot of sense.

The first of these finishing Cat Stance mawashi techniques (facing west), I would suggest, *does* come off the right-side mawashi uke (against the opponent's left arm), though it is easy to see, as I've described above, how the mawashi in Cat Stance might be executed in a number of different ways. Whether the first of these Cat Stance mawashi techniques comes off the left-side mawashi uke or the right-side mawashi uke, in fact, depends on how one executes the head-twisting mawashi. The end result, of course, is the same either way, so one might argue that the bunkai or application is the same; that it's really a matter of individual preference. As I have tried to show, there are only subtle differences in how each of these mawashi techniques is performed, and it should be noted that none of these differences change the bunkai. The only real effect is on how we see the structure of the kata, and there are two important points to keep in mind here: One, that the paired mawashi uke techniques are meant to be taken apart if we are to understand their application; and two, that the mawashi uke in Basic Stance serves as the entry or receiving technique for each of the three series that follows it, forming the core of the first half of the kata.

The Double Punch, Parry, and Left Middle-Level Punch

See figures 3.29–31.

The terms that are generally used to describe the next series of techniques in Suparinpei are poor descriptors, or at best, misleading. In fact, the conventions that have long been used to describe many of the techniques in Okinawan karate, and martial arts in general, more often than not tend to confuse rather than enlighten. The simple act of naming techniques tends to influence how we see a particular movement, but the name we assign any particular technique may be no more than a description of its appearance. A Cat Stance, for example, is a transitional shift to a position where the weight is taken off the leg in order to kick with it. (This might be the front leg in the case of Kururunfa kata, or the rear leg, as we see in the kicking techniques of Saifa kata.) When we call it a "stance," we tend to look for reasons to explain why we would sit in this posture for any length of time. Or we get drawn-out discussions of how low we should sit, or the approximate angle of the bent knee on the supporting leg, or

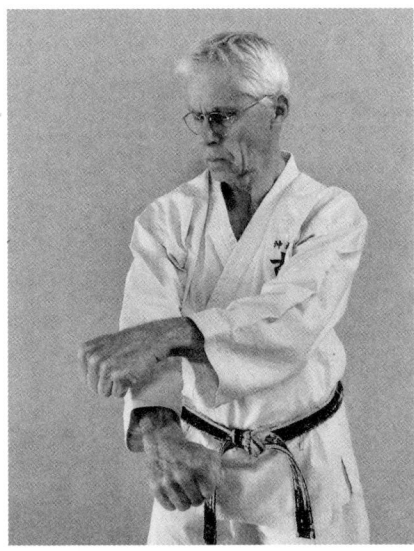

FIGURE 2.26 The right hand pulls
or pushes down as the left hand
"punches" over.

what percentage of weight we should have on each leg. None of this, of course, is really relevant if we see the Cat Stance as a transitional position. It is this intermediary position, the Cat Stance, that is frozen in the still photographs of instructional manuals, including this one.

However, if we were to perform the sequences of kata as they were no doubt meant to be performed in the application of the techniques, these pauses or gaps would disappear. Saifa kata, for example, would show only the movement from shiko dachi in the first sequence of the kata to a right or left kick. And when the Cat Stance is used in the final position of a sequence, as it is at the end of Saifa, it is usually employed as a knee kick (hiza geri)— that is, in the finish posture of the mawashi in Cat Stance, the knee kick has already been employed by the time the final position is shown.

The problem we have with the naming of techniques and how it colors our expectations is widespread, but it is also difficult to avoid. How do you write about any of these techniques without ascribing a name to them? How do you teach without naming them? Shisochin, for instance, has a number of vertical or rising elbow techniques (fig. 2.27). They generally occur at the end of sequences, so they are usually referred to as elbow attacks. Yet because of the techniques that precede each of the rising elbows, it is probably more likely that the technique is a rising palm attack that catches the opponent's chin and thrusts up, twisting the head, as the other hand—the hand that is held in front of the chest and has conventionally been referred to as a guarding hand—holds his head or topknot.

But it is not only the preceding techniques that argue for an interpretation that differs from the conventional elbow attack to the opponent's chest, an attack that seems to occur repeatedly in the kata of Goju-ryu and one that only seems to bolster the notion that karate by nature is a percussive martial art, dominated by kicks and punches. Watching the practice of basics at the beginning of almost any karate class—that part of most classes dominated by the repetitive practice of fundamental blocks, kicks, and punches—would seem to support this view. However, punches and

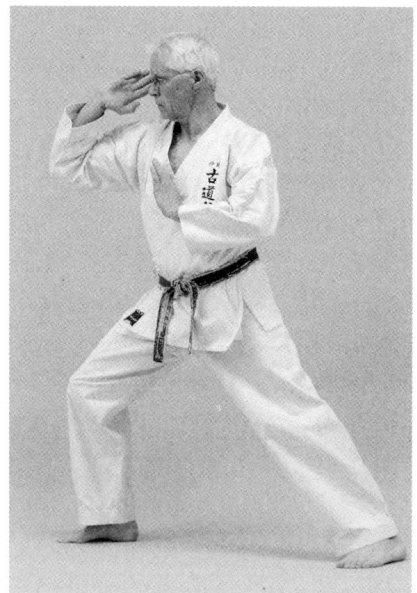

FIGURE 2.27 The rising elbow attacks we see in a performance of Shisochin kata only look like elbow attacks to the opponent's chest.

kicks, by themselves, are not very lethal techniques, and an elbow attack to the opponent's chest, another percussive attack, would not be either. Such an attack, ending a sequence in any of the classical kata, does not fit the tenor of Goju-ryu, and since the technique of what *looks* like a rising elbow attack *does* occur at the end of many sequences, we need to look for another explanation that both fits the movements of kata and the general tenor of the bunkai in the classical subjects.

The same problem occurs in the double punch series we see here in Suparinpei. It may look like a double punch followed by a parry or down block and then a left middle-level punch, but application-wise, I would argue, it is not a double punch nor a right down block nor a left middle-level punch.

The "double punch," of course, can also be found in Sanseiru kata, and it functions in the same way, regardless of the preceding techniques that, at least in appearance, may differ depending on which school of Goju-ryu one subscribes to. In Sanseiru, the double punch technique comes off an

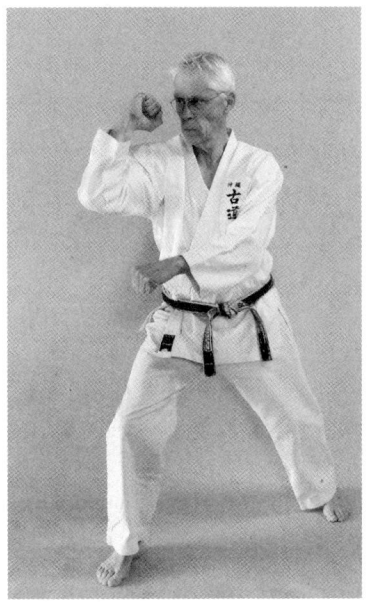

FIGURE 2.28 With the rising elbow attacks in Sanseiru, the "punch" is used to facilitate the head-twisting technique. The left hand has grabbed the hair or top-knot of the opponent early in the sequence.

open-hand controlling technique.[9] In the first instance (moving to the west in Sanseiru kata), the left hand has moved in to control the opponent's chin, while the right hand is brought to the opponent's head or topknot. In the second instance, shown on the opposite side, the hands are reversed. The way that the hands move in Sanseiru helps us to understand the movement of the hands in Suparinpei. In Sanseiru kata, the hand that is on the chin is rotated until it finishes in the higher position, while the hand that is on the head rotates until it finishes in the lower position. The closing of the hands into fists, from the previous open-hand position, signifies the grabbing and holding of the opponent.

In Suparinpei kata, this "double punch" is another technique that comes off the opening mawashi uke and nukite/shuto combination. Just as in the previous case, the mawashi-like technique in Cat Stance, this is a finishing technique that twists the head, a more euphemistic way of describing a neck break. For some, this sort of application is too violent. I have had students and teachers alike, when shown some of these

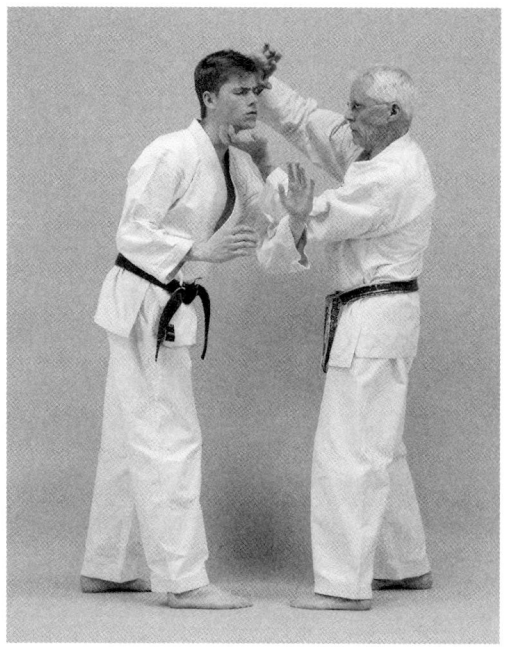

FIGURE 2.29 In the first instance in the Shodokan (Higa) version of Sanseiru, the left hand is brought up to control the opponent's chin while the right hand is used to grab the head or hair. Then, as the defender steps forward, the "double punch" is used to twist the attacker's head.

techniques, tell me, "I can't do that." But this is the nature of Okinawan karate. It was never meant for sport competitions. I would venture to say that virtually all of the finishing techniques one finds in the classical kata attack either the head or neck of the opponent. As a system of self-defense, it is meant to end a life-threatening encounter. Of course, one might vary the strength one uses or the degree to which one uses the various head-twisting techniques, but that doesn't alter the nature of the techniques or change the applications.

In this series, the kata illustrates another way to "finish" the opening mawashi uke sequence. The double punch, parry, and left middle-level punch series, again, like the previous Cat Stance mawashi finishing technique, comes off the *opposite-side* or left mawashi uke and right nukite/shuto. As I mentioned earlier, this is the nukite/shuto that would come off the second of the opening mawashi uke techniques but is not shown in the kata. The double punch series begins from what would be the end position of this left mawashi uke, with the left-hand head grab and right nukite/shuto to the neck. At the beginning of the double punch series, the left hand grabs the head or topknot while the right hand grabs the opponent's chin.

It is possible to execute a credible double punch, parry, and left middle-level punch, the technique that is shown in kata, after either the right mawashi uke or the left mawashi uke. The differences in how one would employ the right arm parry in either case are so subtle that it might seem difficult to determine exactly which of the mawashi uke techniques is meant to be used with the double punch, parry, and left middle-level punch. In fact, much of it depends simply on how and when (or whether) one employs the 90-degree or 180-degree turns, implied in the application of each. I would suggest, however, that the stronger argument is that the left mawashi uke along with the right nukite/shuto is indicated here, since this is the side used with the following angular shiko dachi technique, the third of the finishing techniques shown in the first half of the kata.

The initial head twist is *executed on the turn*—this is important to remember—using what we call the "double punch." Just as we see in Sanseiru kata, the hand that is on the chin is rotated until it finishes in the higher position, while the hand that is on the head rotates until it finishes in the lower position. The "parry" or "down block" with the right hand is used to pull or push the attacker's head down. And the left middle-level "punch," the hand that is grabbing the head or hair, is thrust out, over the right wrist or forearm, further twisting the opponent's neck. It is also interesting to note that when the "double punch" is employed with a 90-degree turn or a 180-degree turn, after *either* the left or the right mawashi uke, the right "parry" and left "punch" is still the same—that is, the technique we see in kata may be employed with either the left or right mawashi uke.

In some schools, the double punch technique is done with a slight sinking of the body. The knees bend and the body lowers as the turn is made and the hands are pulled in. Then the knees straighten a little as the turn completes and the hands are thrust out. The preservation of this kind of movement in the kata was no doubt meant to add power to the manipulation of the opponent. After all, one is attempting to twist the head of an opponent that may be attached to a sizable body.

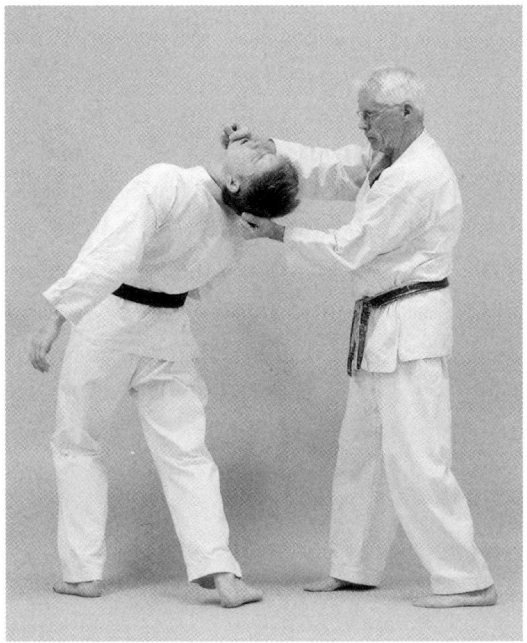

FIGURE 2.30 In the double punch technique of Suparinpei kata, the left hand is on the attacker's head and the right hand has seized the opponent's chin. This is the same as the second instance of the double punch technique in the Shodokan (Higa) version of Sanseiru, facing east, prior to the final technique of the kata.

It is interesting to note, though it is of little actual consequence, the degree to which the performance speed or tempo of these techniques in kata seems to vary, and it highlights, I suppose, how attuned to nuance and minutia we have become. Each of these subtle differences in performance seems to raise the specter of hidden meaning, and speculation about what may only be idiosyncratic preferences creeps into these discussions of possible applications. When we see the entire sequence of movements performed with speed and a considerable use of force, we assume that the movements show percussive, closed-fist attacks—that is, an actual double punch to the opponent's torso, followed by a parrying or blocking motion with the right forearm, finishing with a left punch to the opponent's chest. Sometimes the tempo of the three techniques of this series varies so much—from a slow parrying motion, showing the use of dynamic tension, to a quick explosive punch—that it seems to suggest the countering of multiple attacks from the opponent.

However, the speed at which each of these techniques is executed has less to do with the speed we would associate with the percussive impact of a punch than it does with the strength one would employ in the twisting motion associated with the application and how we imagine that. In other words, the double punch here, used as the initial head-twisting technique, should not be executed with the same speed and power (or, obviously, intent) as one would use in executing an awase tsuki (combined or "u" punch) or a *nihon tsuki* (double punch). Each of the techniques of this series—the double punch, parry, and left middle-level punch—should be executed with the speed and power one might use in manipulating the *kongoken* (iron oval weight). It is always worth remembering that in addition to manipulating the opponent's head, there is likely a two-hundred-pound body attached to it. In application, the only real consideration that dictates the amount of force or speed is the mass and inertia of the opponent. In the first of these techniques, the double punch, we are holding the attacker's head, pushing forward to twist the head and disrupt the opponent's balance, a common theme in Suparinpei and also in many of the other classical kata.

One further note to remember when one is practicing these techniques in kata is that there is really no need, if one is executing the application correctly, to draw the left fist back into a chambered position; the left "fist," which is holding onto the opponent's head or hair, need only be pushed out and down to twist the attacker's neck, completing the sequence.

Shiko Dachi (Horse Stance) to the Four Corners

See figures 3.32–34.

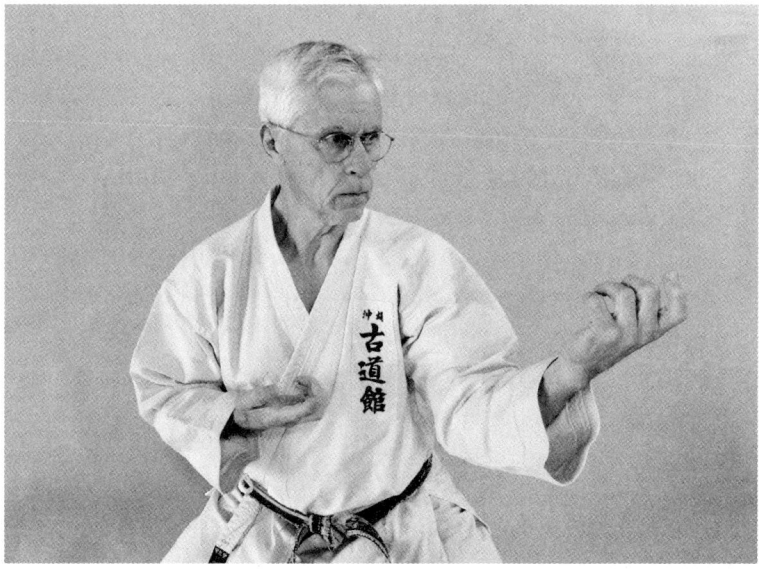

FIGURE 2.31 Stepping into shiko dachi along the forward angle is yet another technique used in Suparinpei to control the opponent.

This is the last of the combinations of the first half meant to be attached to the opening mawashi uke sequence and may present the most difficult challenge to those trying to decipher the movements of kata and come up with a viable application. Something about the angles is reminiscent of Seiunchin kata: they both move in, using Horse Stance, along the ordinal compass points, with hand movements that look like down blocks or lower-level strikes. To add to the confusion, some Okinawan schools appear to use a single-knuckle fist with the beginning shiko dachi, while others use an open hand or partially closed hand. Some teachers have even suggested that this latter hand position implies that the kata was originally a *rokushaku bo* (six-foot staff) kata, with the partially closed hand meant to imply that the practitioner is holding a *bo*. Everything is possible, as the saying goes; however, not everything is logical or provides one with the best answer.

Some others have reasoned that this posture is nothing more than a kamae or kind of en garde position—that there is no intrinsic application to be found here. This may be due in part to the change in direction, since directional changes, at least in Suparinpei, seem to be used to indicate the beginning of a new sequence, at least in the second half of the kata. Although it is not so difficult to find a kind of application that not only follows the movements of the kata but also conforms to most of our expectations of block and punch bunkai. One need only imagine an attacker stepping in with a left punch as the defender steps back at an angle, using the left forearm to intercept the attacker's punch. Then, as the defender's left hand turns to guard and push against the attacker's elbow, the defender shifts into a left-foot-forward Front Stance, attacking with the single-knuckle punch. In the following step into a right shiko dachi to the corner, the defender continues with a lower attack.

In fact, it is very possible that the finishing counterattack in this shiko dachi angle technique from Suparinpei is the same finishing downward forearm strike that we see in the angle sequence from Seiunchin kata (the second sequence) or the angle sequence in Seipai kata (fourth sequence). The problem we encounter in trying to interpret these movements is that there seems to be a technique between the two shiko dachi stances in Suparinpei. We generally shift into a left-foot-forward Front Stance from the first Horse Stance, and the hands, at least when we try to capture the movements in still photographs, suggest the need to provide some additional explanation (see fig. 2.32). However, if one were to move from the first Horse Stance to the second Horse Stance, without pausing, then there is very little noticeable change to the movements we ordinarily practice. Perhaps we have overstylized the movements of kata, looking for a single-knuckle punch or a head twist where there is simply a downward forearm strike.

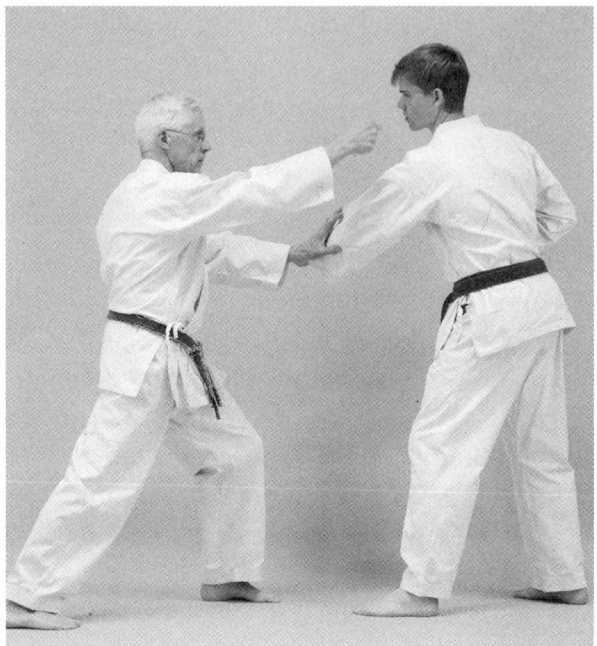

FIGURE 2.32 A conventional block/punch explanation for this shiko dachi angle technique in Suparinpei.

It would be tempting to teach either (or both) of these applications to beginners since they are relatively safe ways to train the movements. The problem, however, with teaching what some describe as different levels of application (bunkai) is that these alternative explanations tend to color the way we "see" kata, making it even more difficult to understand, and put into practice, some of the principles these movements are meant to illustrate.

And there are certainly a number of other problems with this sort of block and punch explanation, not least of which is the notion that the opponent is required to hold his punch out while the defender counterattacks. It may seem to work in the dojo against a compliant partner, but it is doubtful that it would work in a more realistic situation. Then, of course, there is the question that the stance itself raises. The Horse Stance or shiko dachi is a stable stance, used in order to bring the opponent down or to attack when the opponent has been taken to the ground. In the classical kata of Goju-ryu, we don't find it being used in conjunction with intercepting an opponent's punch.

The best clue to the application of the shiko dachi series is probably the structure of the first half of Suparinpei kata. The structure suggests, once again, that each of these three series of techniques should be seen as a continuation of the opening mawashi uke series, and since this certainly seems to be the case with the first two series—the mawashi in Cat Stance and the "double punch"—there is no reason to believe that this would not include the third series as well.

Adding to the difficulty of actually "seeing" each of these applications is the fact that the latter two of these techniques come off the opposite-side mawashi uke and nukite/shuto—again, the side that is only partially shown in kata. Using the complete left-side mawashi uke (against the opponent's right arm) and right nukite/shuto, the defender's left hand would already have seized the opponent's hair or topknot. (We should imagine the defender facing west at this point in the kata.) As the defender steps with the right foot to the northwest angle into shiko dachi, with the attention directed at the southeast corner—the first of these shiko dachi angle techniques shown in the kata—the opponent is pulled forward, off balance, and the head is twisted in such a way that the chin is exposed or facing up (see fig. 2.33). In the next move, the defender would bring his or her right hand out to attack (or push) the opponent's chin (see fig. 2.34), stepping into a right-foot-forward shiko dachi as both arms are brought down and out (see fig. 3.34), twisting the opponent's head or neck, or, alternatively, attacking the opponent's neck with the dropping right forearm, as we see in Seiunchin kata.

One should note the similarity, however subtle it may appear at first, between this movement into the left shiko dachi, with the defender's left hand holding the opponent's hair or topknot, and the "core" technique of Sanseiru kata. After the opening sequence of Sanseiru, the kata turns into a south-facing Basic Stance with the left arm held in front of the body in what appears to be a middle-level chest block. This is followed by a front kick and right elbow technique. The sequence is repeated two more times on the same side—showing a 90-degree turn and a 180-degree turn to the left. When these techniques are connected to the initial arm-folding or scissoring technique of the kata, we see something similar to what we have illustrated in the shiko dachi angle techniques of Suparinpei. After the initial arm-folding technique of Sanseiru, the left hand grabs the opponent's hair or topknot. This is followed by a right kick. The "elbow" technique, executed in a right zenkutsu dachi, is the result or end position after the defender pushes up on the opponent's chin with the right hand while pulling back on the opponent's hair with the left hand, effectively twisting the head.

One of the principles we can note in this shiko dachi series from Suparinpei is the use of off-line movement. But we can also see what seems to be a rather simple explanation for the different hand positions one sees in various schools. The open hand, of course, merely represents that this is an open-hand technique, not a punching technique. The fist or half-fist, or open hand with the fingers slightly curled in, all represent the grabbing techniques employed in the application.

The shiko dachi angle technique that we see in kata, with the left hand up and the right hand held in front of the chest, is most likely meant to come off the initial left-side mawashi uke and right nukite—pushing in against and grabbing the opponent's right arm—as I have described it. However, one can also imagine the same left shiko dachi angle technique being used with the right-side mawashi uke and left nukite. In that case, the opponent's chin would be in the left hand and the defender's right hand would be grabbing the hair or topknot. The same angle step to the northwest (in the case of the first of these angle techniques shown in kata) would be used, with the attacker to the west. The following technique, stepping through into a right shiko dachi, would also be slightly different but equally effective and in line with the general tenor of the kata. The major difference in applying the technique this way would be that the hands would need to be a lot closer together in the initial step into shiko dachi—what would seem to be a bit of a departure from a strict interpretation of kata movement—and the defender would not pause, even the slightest bit, in the execution of the technique. Of course, if one is strictly adhering to the movements of kata in the interpretation of technique (bunkai), then it seems more likely that the shiko dachi angle techniques we see in Suparinpei require the use of the left-side mawashi uke and right nukite.

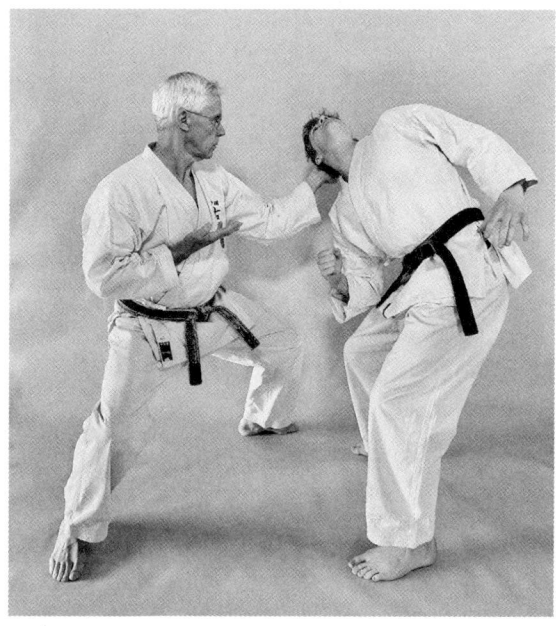

FIGURE 2.33 The first shiko dachi technique off the opposite-side mawashi uke and nukite/shuto.

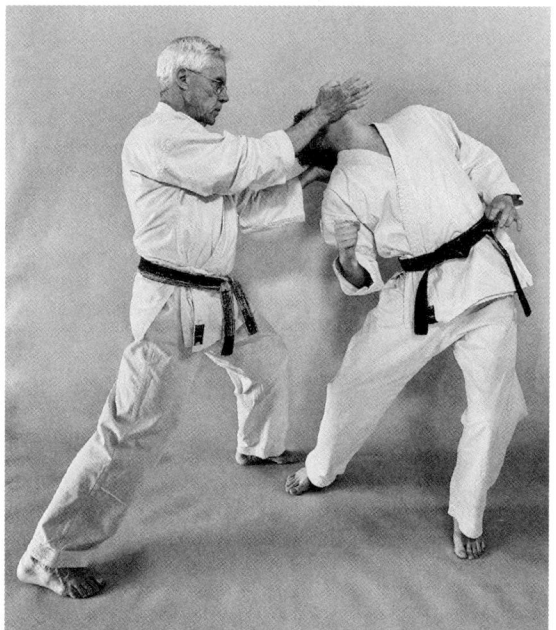

FIGURE 2.34 Shifting forward to attack the chin and twist the head as the defender begins to step through into a right-foot-forward shiko dachi.

The First Complete Sequence

See figures 3.35–42.

Much like Seisan, to which it is no doubt closely related, the first half of Suparinpei kata comprises somewhat fragmented techniques, while the second half of the kata demonstrates complete bunkai sequences—that is, sequences composed of entry techniques, bridging techniques, and finishing techniques. And, like the earlier series of techniques in the first half of the kata, these second-half sequences illustrate close-in fighting strategies, beginning from a clinch, a two-handed grab, or any posture where the opponent has closed in with both arms up.

The first complete sequence of the kata shows the defender stepping forward with the left foot, facing the original front of the kata, as the left arm moves in a clockwise, semicircular fashion with the palm or forearm

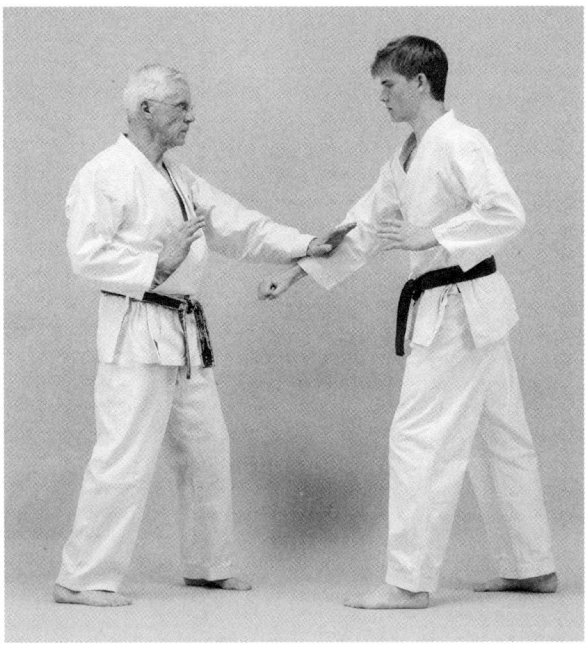

FIGURE 2.35 The first entry step and block of the first full sequence. From a clinch, this is the movement associated with the defender's outside arm.

pressing down and finishing in the gedan position. The right foot then steps forward into Basic Stance with the right arm moving up in a clockwise semicircular fashion with the palm facing forward. The forward motion that accompanies the circular blocking motions should be viewed as an integral aspect of the sequence—that is, one should always consider that the movement of the feet shown in kata is as important as the movement of the hands. In this case, the stepping serves to press or unbalance the opponent, pushing him onto his heels and into a defensive, rather than offensive, posture.

It should also be noted that most of the blocking motions of Goju-ryu are circular in nature, rather than linear, percussive, or meeting force with force. Most of these blocking motions move around the opponent's attack or redirect the opponent's attack along the path of least resistance.

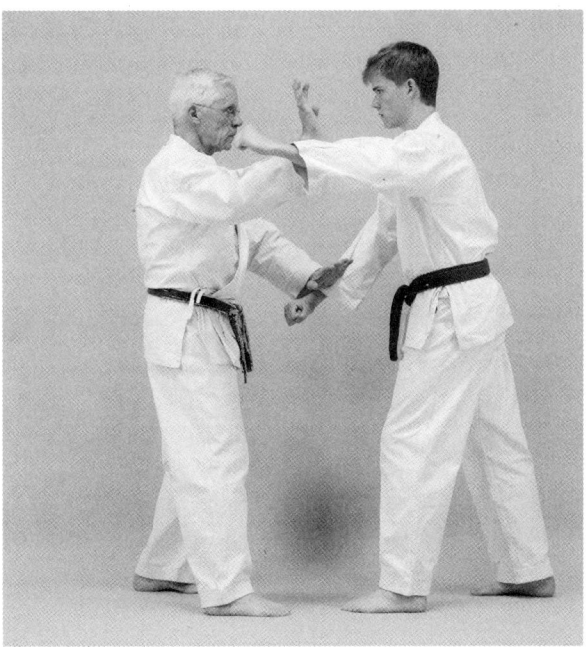

FIGURE 2.36 The second entry step and block of the first full sequence. From a clinch, this is the movement associated with the defender's inside arm.

Therefore, most of the "blocking" (the receiving or uke techniques) that we see in Goju-ryu seem to take little effort. Additionally, the forearms should be used to block or intercept the opponent's attack, rather than the hands.

For some, the two-hand, outside-inside entry technique seen here in this first sequence—using the left semicircular down block and the right semicircular rising block—will be reminiscent of what is often referred to as the "sun and moon" block found in the Shodokan (Higa) version of Seisan kata, though here in the first full sequence of Suparinpei it is shown on the opposite side from what we see in Seisan.

It is called the sun and moon block ostensibly because the circular motion of one hand is a bit larger than the circular motion of the other hand, or perhaps because they seem to chase each other like the sun and moon rising and setting on the horizon. As the technique is shown in Seisan kata, each hand describes two partial circles. (This is actually an important concept that shows up in the last sequence of Suparinpei kata.)

Other schools do not use the sun and moon block in the opening section of Seisan kata—the front-facing series of three techniques, each

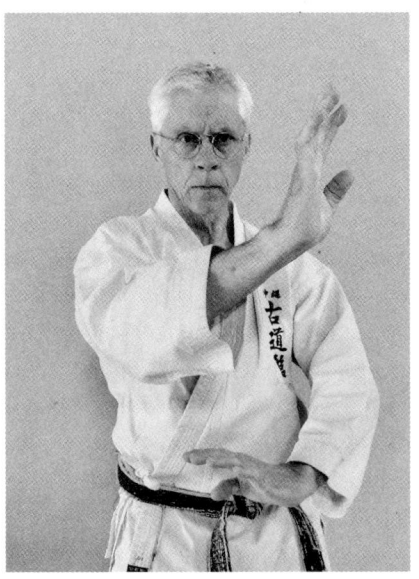

FIGURE 2.37 The "sun and moon" block is difficult to capture in a still photograph, but it looks similar to the open-hand chest blocks that we see in Shisochin and the Gekisai kata. However, in Seisan kata, the sun and moon block is done higher, at the jodan level, and each hand circles twice—which, interestingly, is how it is used in the last sequence of Suparinpei kata.

repeated three times and ending in a grab and down side kick. Rather, they will show what appears to be a series of three rising palm strikes—first with the left, then with the right, and then again with the left. Though these two versions of the Seisan technique may appear to be different—the first one, the Shodokan sun and moon block, looks like a block because of its circular nature, while the rising palm strike looks like an attack because of its more linear nature—they may actually function the same way. The only thing that may really differ in how they are applied is the angle of the arc used to intercept the opponent's attacking arms.

It's curious that this technique—the double-arm entry technique of this first complete sequence in Suparinpei kata—moving as it does to "open" the opponent, seems to differ so much in principle from the opening mawashi uke series in the first half, which moves to the *outside* of the attacker. Here, as in each of the subsequent combinations or sequences in Suparinpei, the defender is moving to the *inside*, or more precisely the inside of the opponent's two arms.

On a related note, this entry technique that we see in each of the sequences in the second half of Suparinpei—one of three entry techniques

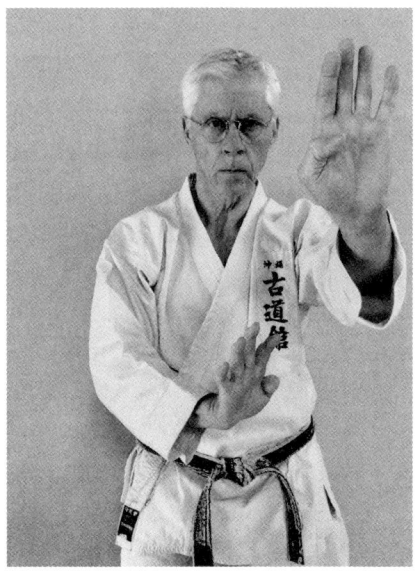

FIGURE 2.38 If we imagine, as is probably the case, that originally the bunkai for each of these techniques was the same, then the downward motion of the hands in these rising palm strikes is as important as the upward movement.

in the kata and the entry or receiving technique for each of the three complete bunkai sequences—may also help us to understand the function of the four open-palm techniques we see in the middle of Shisochin kata, techniques that have conventionally been interpreted as open-hand lower blocks with one hand and palm strikes with the other hand. While it is certainly possible that this is a single technique, independent of any initial entry technique or subsequent finishing techniques, given the sequential structure of most other techniques and kata in Goju-ryu, it seems at least as likely that the open-palm techniques of Shisochin function as an entry technique similar to each of the open-hand entries we see in the three sequences in the second half of Suparinpei kata.

When we see the sun and moon block used in Seisan kata, it is most obvious in the second full sequence of the kata—the sequence that moves from west to east, from Basic Stance to shiko dachi. Coincidentally, the second sequence of Seisan begins the same as the last sequence of Suparinpei. But a part of the sun and moon block begins the first and third sequences of Seisan kata also. And this is where an understanding of Suparinpei becomes extremely helpful. To begin the first sequence of Seisan kata, we turn 180 degrees to the south. Some schools will make this turn using a right circular block, ending in the down position, while attacking with a left straight-arm palm strike. If we were to apply the martial principle that it is always better to move to the outside of the opponent's attack, then the stepping pattern of the kata would suggest that the attacker is stepping in from the west with a left punch. By turning, we are side-stepping the attack, blocking with the right and attacking with the left palm (see fig. 2.39). Other schools, however, make this turn with a right circular down block and a left circular rising block, both hands open and moving in a counterclockwise direction, though somewhat larger than the open-hand blocking motions that we see in the middle of Shisochin kata or the Gekisai kata.

Interestingly, the first of these methods—blocking with the right and attacking with a left palm strike—implies a number of different things: The turns in kata suggest stepping off line, to the outside of the opponent's attack. The opponent is attacking with a punch, and the defender

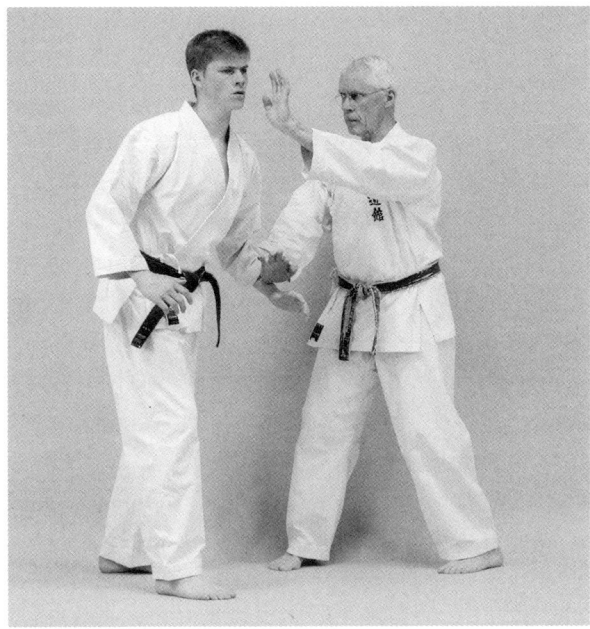

FIGURE 2.39 Using the straight-arm palm strike in the
first sequence of Seisan kata implies that the opponent
is attacking from the west with a left punch.

is responding similarly with an open-palm strike to the face. And lastly,
it seems to call into question the seemingly thematic connection that the
opening series of techniques we see in the first half of the kata are based
on a grappling or clinch scenario, though it is certainly feasible that the
kata is showing both possibilities.

The second method, however, where we are turning to the south with
two circular blocking techniques—one dropping and the other rising—
suggests that this is an inside technique against a two-handed attack,
whether that is two punches, or a two-handed grab, or the opponent is
standing in the clinch or grappling posture (see fig. 2.40).

The idea that the entry or receiving techniques we see in the second
half of Suparinpei move to the inside of the opponent's defenses suggests
that Suparinpei may, in fact, illustrate a more complete self-defense strat-
egy than any of the other classical kata of Goju-ryu. The entry techniques

preserved in Suparinpei show movement to both the inside and the out-side of the opponent's attack, as well as responses to a two-armed clinch or grappling scenario or a punching attack with either one or both hands.

This is where an understanding of Suparinpei may be helpful, because this technique in the first complete sequence of Suparinpei is obviously an *inside* technique, though it is executed on the opposite side from Seisan kata. (Because this first complete sequence of Suparinpei kata is shown on the opposite side from the second and third sequences, even though the entry techniques are the same, and there is no stepping off line or change of direction, it seems a strong confirmation that the entry techniques of all three sequences are meant to be seen as inside techniques, reinforcing the notion that thematically we are exploring close-in or clinch scenarios in Suparinpei rather than the more conventional block/punch attacks and counters.) So one might ask, though for some it may seem a bit outside the purview of this discussion of Suparinpei, is one method wrong and the other right in our analysis of Seisan? Interestingly, the bunkai for the rest of the first sequence in Seisan is essentially the same regardless of

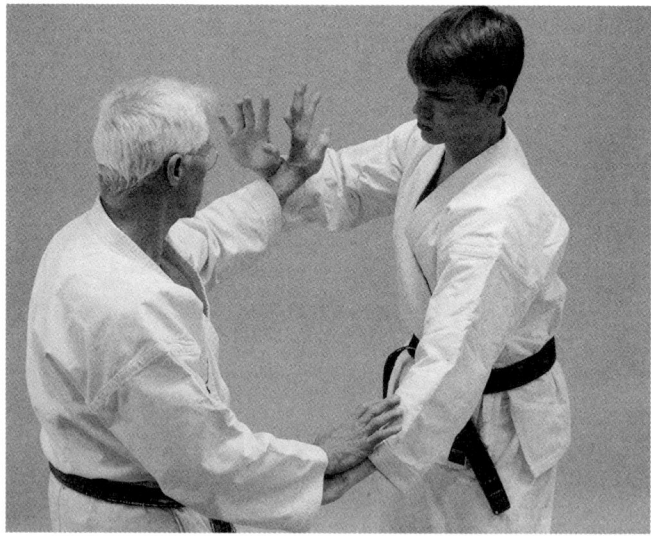

FIGURE 2.40 The entry technique of the first sequence of Seisan kata as an inside technique or against a clinch.

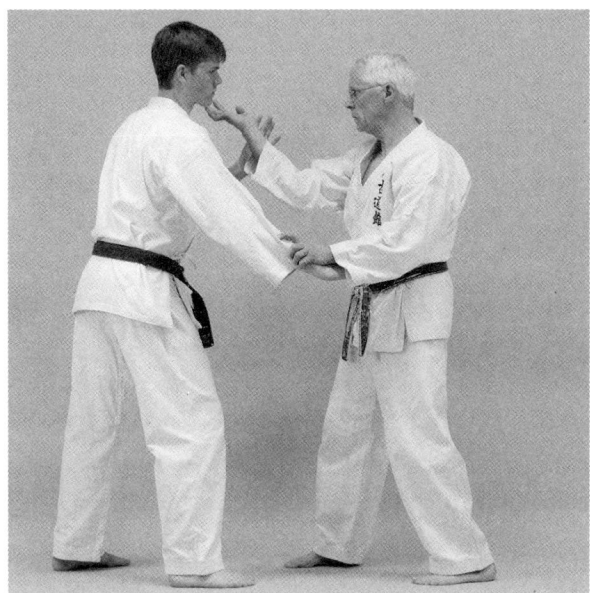

FIGURE 2.41 Stepping forward into the palm-up technique from the first sequence of Seisan kata. Coincidentally, this is the same entry and attack we see in the second complete sequence of Suparinpei kata.

which entry method is used. So I suppose it all depends on how strongly one might feel the connection between Seisan kata and Suparinpei kata is. Personally, I believe that Seisan and Suparinpei are so closely related that an understanding of one helps in our understanding of the other.

That being said, Suparinpei continues from here, stepping into a left-foot-forward stance—in some schools this third step is into Basic Stance and in other schools, notably the Shodokan (Higa) lineage, into a Front Stance—with the left arm up, palm forward, and right arm down, wrist bent, with the fingers pointing forward (see fig. 3.37).

This is one of the few techniques in Suparinpei that is done differently in different schools of Okinawan Goju-ryu. Most of the time, the differences we see in the performance of the classical kata are generally insignificant or superficial, often showing only what seem to be idiosyncratic preferences in timing or rhythm. However, the semicircular blocking motion that accompanies the step into a left-foot-forward Basic Stance that is shown in some schools of Goju-ryu, reminiscent of the open-hand chest blocks we see in the Gekisai kata, seems to me difficult to justify, particularly in the context of the techniques that come immediately before this technique and immediately after it. If it is in fact meant to accompany the initial left downward semicircular block and right rising semicircular block, stepping into a right-foot-forward Basic Stance, then the effect of this second blocking technique would, if successful, control the attacker's left arm and turn the opponent around. The subsequent right front kick, right elbow attack, and neck break would then be delivered to the opponent's back. And while this is certainly a possible explanation, it seems a bit unrealistic, requiring the opponent to "hold" his left attacking arm out long enough for the defender to manipulate it and turn the opponent. A more likely explanation, I think, is that the circular motion of this left open-hand block, stepping into the left-foot-forward Basic Stance, has been exaggerated or at the very least homogenized to make it look like the familiar open-hand chest block or *chudan hiki uke*. If, however, the movement of the left open hand is more linear, or if the left hand is not brought under the right elbow or forearm but simply brought around in contact with the opponent's neck, it would function very much like the palm strike in zenkutsu dachi that we see in the Shodokan (Higa) version.

In application, it is difficult to say whether the right hand has been used to grab and pull the opponent's left arm, though I suspect it has, since this would make sense within the context of the sequence and would just be good technique. (Interestingly, this would be a same-side grab with the defender's right hand blocking and then grabbing the attacker's left arm. We might, therefore, look at each of the receiving techniques of Saifa kata as counters or responses to the same-side grab techniques that begin each of the sequences in the second half of Suparinpei kata.) The difficulty is that Suparinpei seems to differ from some of the lower classical kata in the Goju canon in that a grabbing hand is not always shown by a technique that either opens from a closed-fist position or closes from an open-hand position. For example, in this position from the first sequence of Seiunchin kata (fig. 2.42), the right hand has gone from an open hand to a closed hand because it is grabbing and twisting the opponent's hair or topknot.

In reality, particularly since it would seem that the classical kata of Goju-ryu probably derive from different sources, there isn't really a uniform rule in kata to indicate where or when the defender is grabbing the opponent. The sequences of Suparinpei kata have a number of places where a grab of the opponent is not only possible but, based on logic, highly probable.

In any case, the Shodokan version of this technique looks very much like the four-directional palm strikes in Shisochin kata, and whether this technique in Suparinpei kata is used as an initial strike to the head of the opponent or merely a way to get the left hand in a position behind the opponent's head in preparation for the next technique (or both), it is followed almost immediately with a right front kick *(mae geri)*(fig. 2.45).

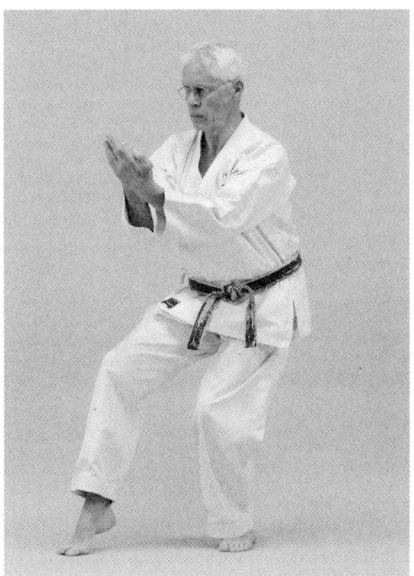

FIGURE 2.42 The closed right hand has grabbed and begun twisting the opponent's hair, while the left hand controls the chin.

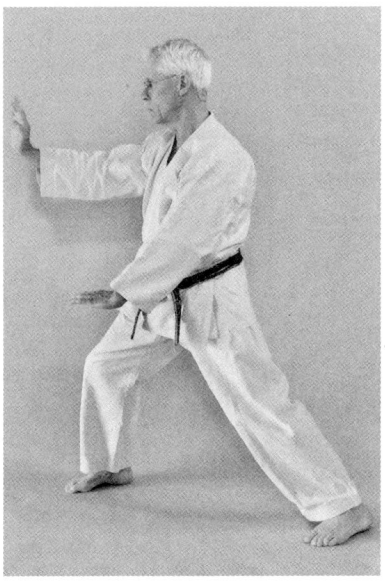

FIGURE 2.43 This open-hand technique, one of four in Shisochin kata, looks very much like the palm technique in the Shodokan (Higa) version of Suparinpei.

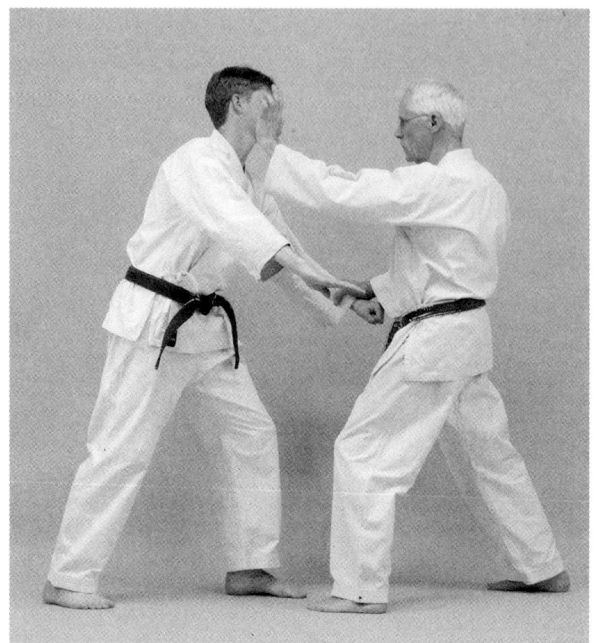

FIGURE 2.44 Using the left palm to attack and the right open hand to pull the opponent in and down.

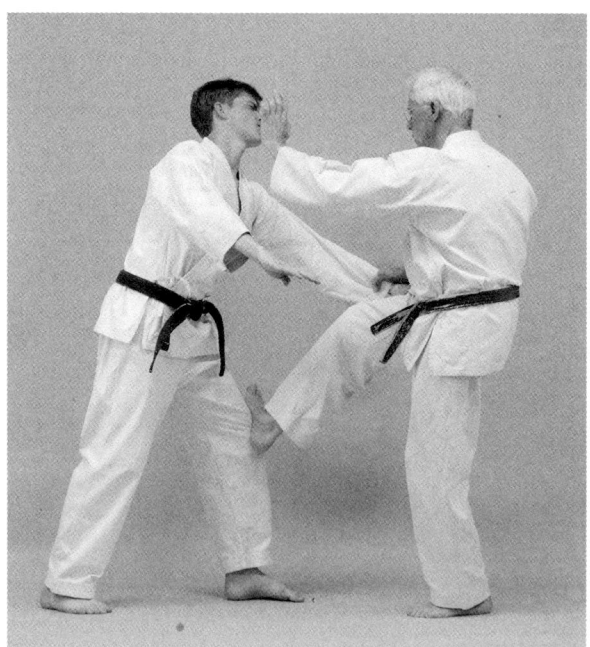

FIGURE 2.45 The front kick is used to bring the opponent's head down.

The primary purpose of the front kick is to bring the opponent's head in and down, as the defender's foot is planted in a right-foot-forward shiko dachi. Once that is accomplished, the left hand serves to bring the head into a horizontal attack with the right elbow. This is one of the few elbow techniques we see in Goju-ryu. The vertical "elbow" strikes that characterize the conventional interpretation of certain techniques in Shisochin, Sanseiru, and Kururunfa are more than likely head-twisting techniques, where the right hand that accompanies the rising "elbow" attack pushes the opponent's chin up as the left hand controls the opponent's head.

It may be important to note at this point that the right elbow is not used to attack the opponent's ribs, even though by all appearances the technique is executed at that height in kata—that is, what we see in kata is that the defender is already in Horse Stance as he or she brings the right elbow across the chest, horizontally, to meet his or her left hand. Though that may be the conventional bunkai or analysis of this technique, what such interpretations fail to take into account is the reaction of the opponent to the

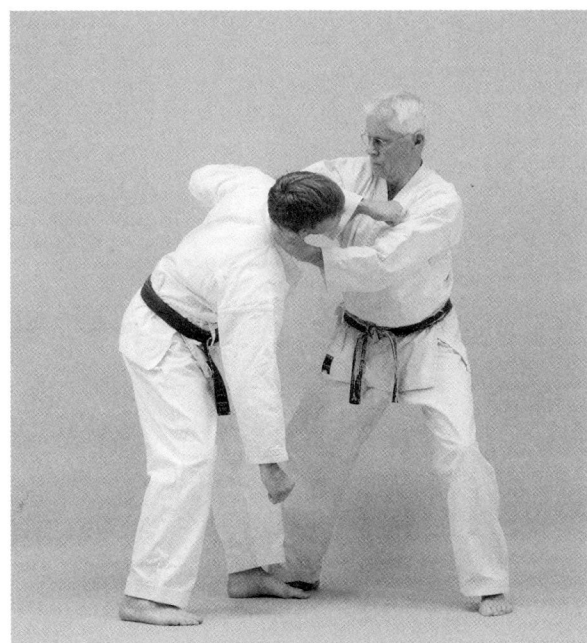

FIGURE 2.46 The left hand controls the opponent's head as the right elbow is used to attack.

techniques that precede it. This is often the case, and one of the pitfalls we encounter in trying to figure out what exactly is going on in kata. In other words, if you kick the opponent—provided your kick is effective and has the intended effect—then it will necessarily bring the opponent forward and down. You drop into Horse Stance to attack the head, which is now at that level. Some people, of course, will object to the elbow technique being dependent on bringing the head down. "What do you do if your kick does not bring the opponent's head down or if it's off target?" they ask. And, of course, the simple answer is, you do something else (see appendix A for an example of this). Each subsequent technique of a given sequence in kata is based on the effect of the techniques that precede it.

The next technique in this sequence shows the right arm unfolding, with the forearm now more or less vertical rather than horizontal, and the left open hand rotated vertically along the side of the right forearm (see fig. 3.40).

This is not really a technique, though it is often thought to be an *uraken* or back-fist strike, but rather a quick repositioning of the right arm in

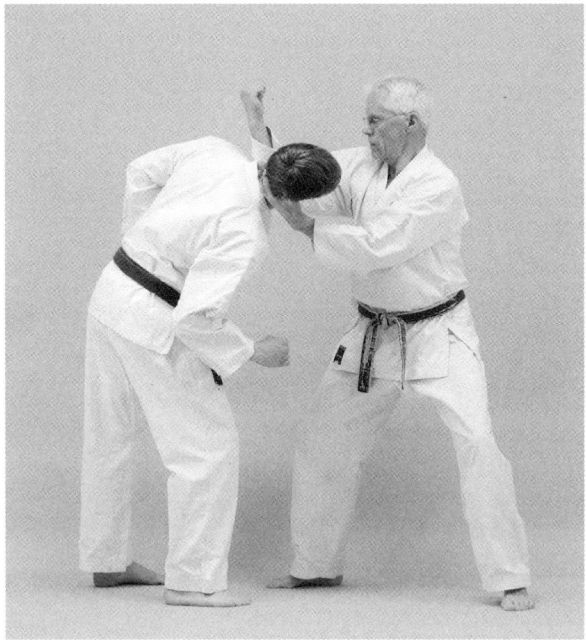

FIGURE 2.47 The right arm unfolds until it is along the left side of the attacker's head.

order to grab the opponent by the back of the head or by the hair. We see a similar movement being used in the fourth sequence of Seiunchin kata in order to bring the opponent's head down to attack with a dropping forearm in Horse Stance. In fact, the uraken or back-fist strike is probably another technique that is missing from the classical kata of Goju-ryu. Based on the structure and sequence of moves we see in each of the kata— conventionally the back-fist strike is said to occur in Saifa, Seiunchin, Seipai, and Suparinpei—the striking surface is most likely the forearm or the elbow rather than the back of the fist. This is also one of the reasons why the practice of *kote kitae* or arm conditioning is important.

In Suparinpei, as the right hand opens to grab the opponent by the hair or back of the head, the left open hand slides up the right forearm until it reaches the opponent's chin or, in the case of the actual application, the left hand slides around the head to grab the opponent's chin (fig. 2.50). The right hand then *pulls* forcefully as the left hand *pushes out* with equal force, effectively twisting the attacker's head and breaking the neck.

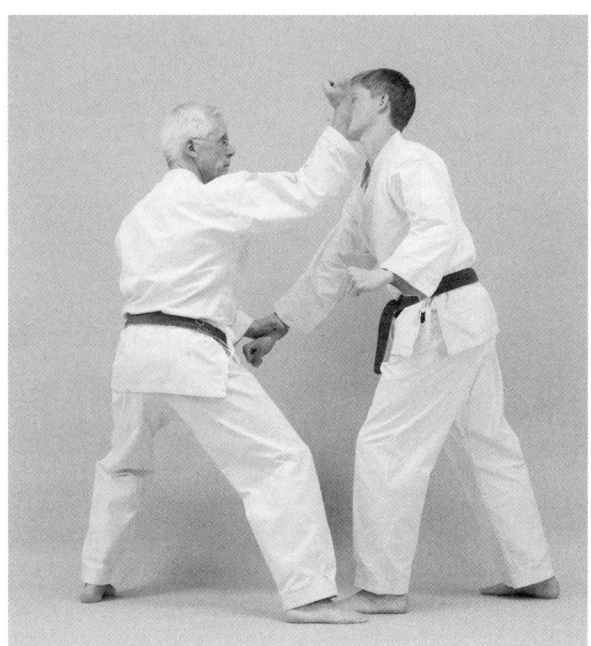

FIGURE 2.48 After the initial counterattack in the fourth sequence of Sei-unchin kata, the right arm is in a position to bring the opponent's head down as the defender steps back to attack the neck with the left *gedan uke* or *gedan barai* (or forearm attack).

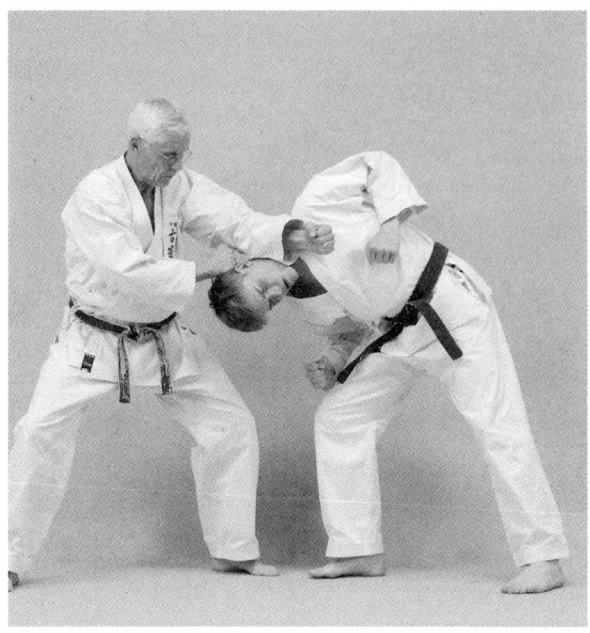

FIGURE 2.49 Stepping back into shiko dachi to finish with the downward forearm strike in Seiunchin.

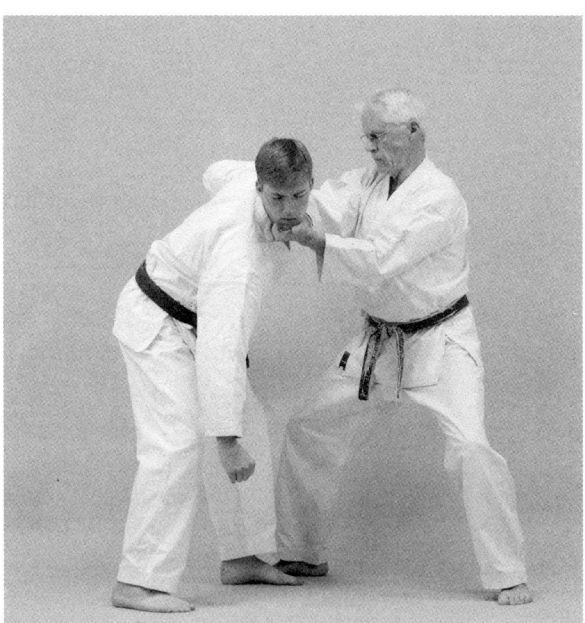

FIGURE 2.50 The head-twisting or neck-break technique from the first complete sequence of Suparinpei.

I should emphasize, I suppose, that if one is interested in the study of traditional karate, one may have to let go of certain tendencies that have taken hold in many dojo due, I suspect, to the advent of sport karate. One of these is that less violent techniques have been substituted and have become the conventional standards—the uraken, in my opinion, being one example. Another is that the rhythm of kata has been altered, perhaps for the simple reason that when slowed down and punctuated, it makes for a better show. The first sequence of Suparinpei kata, in other words, should be performed without any gaps or pauses, from beginning to end. At times, we are working against the imagined inertia of the opponent's body so the techniques will necessarily be somewhat slower, but the flow of the techniques should be continuous, without the staccato movement that one often sees in the performance of kata before an audience or judges armed with score cards.

The Second Complete Sequence

See figures 3.43–48.

The second complete sequence of Suparinpei kata begins with a turn to the south with the same "blocking" or, more properly, the same uke (receiving) technique we see in the first sequence of Seisan kata. And since both of these kata begin with the double-arm kamae posture—both arms held up in front of the body, like the opening posture of Sanchin—the suggestion is that each of these entry techniques works to the inside of the opponent's clinch or grappling posture. This is essentially the same receiving technique that we see in the first complete sequence of the kata but on the opposite side.

Some schools, however, follow the right arm circular block in both Suparinpei and Seisan with what appears to be a left open-hand palm strike. This combination seems to be similar to what we see in Shisochin kata, except in this case the left arm is not brought up in an arcing motion but thrust straight out. The stance, of course, is also higher, as both Seisan and Suparinpei utilize Basic Stance instead of Front Stance. And while this technique may also be used to move to the inside of the opponent's clinch, I suspect it may have been thought of as a block and attack against a left punch from an attacker stepping in from the west, the defender stepping off line in order to avoid the attack while blocking with the right arm circular block (see fig. 2.39).

The rest of the bunkai could certainly be adapted to fit this scenario, but one of the problems is that the open-hand attack to the opponent's face may have the unwanted consequence of pushing the attacker away rather than gaining control of him or her. And in any case, Suparinpei seems to be exploring the idea of moving to the inside in a close-in confrontation.

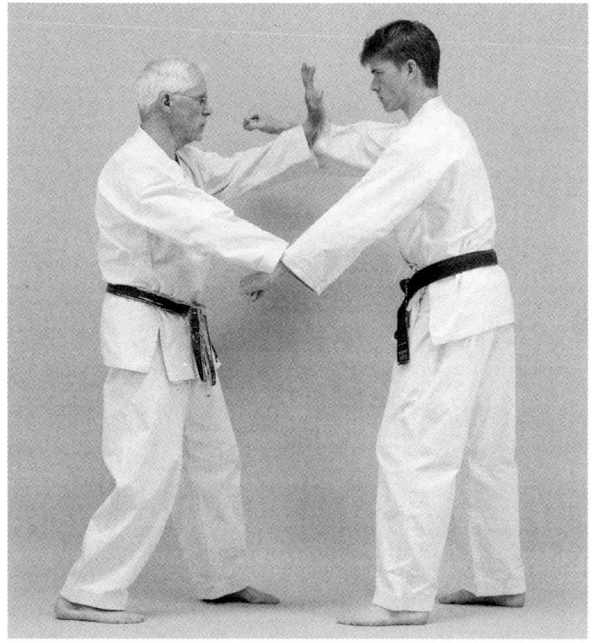

FIGURE 2.51 If we imagine this sequence beginning from something other than a grappling position—where the mawashi uke would come into play—it might be something like the en garde posture. The defender holds both hands up in a defensive posture, one hand slightly higher than the other. As the attacker moves in, the defender steps back. The defender's right arm is brought down to cover the attacker's left arm, while the defender's left arm is brought up to cover the attacker's right arm, effectively moving inside the opponent's defenses to continue the counterattack.

The other possibility, of course, is that the left straight-arm palm strike may be used as a *tsuki uke* or combination block-attack—that is, not stepping off line but turning to face the attacker and simultaneously blocking and attacking with the same hand. But again, even this combination block-attack may not control the attacker.

If, as many schools perform these arm motions, we turn to the south and use both arms in a *circular* fashion, on the other hand, then there is no question, it would seem to me, that this is intended as an inside technique, just as we see in the first complete sequence of Suparinpei. Further, the left rising arm is positioned to grab and control the opponent's right wrist as it is brought down in the next move, when the right foot steps forward. And, of course, as an inside technique it is easy to see how this entry technique might be employed with the initial mawashi uke that we see at the beginning of the kata.

Each of the remaining sequences in Suparinpei, in fact, comes off a turn to the left, with the second and third sequences showing the same side entry technique as Seisan—the right arm circling down and the left arm circling up—but the opposite side from the *first* sequence of Suparinpei. Once again, it may be of interest to note here that there are obvious similarities between the sequences of Seisan kata and Suparinpei kata. This second sequence of Suparinpei shows marked similarities to the first sequence of Seisan kata, and the second sequence of Seisan is very similar to the last sequence of Suparinpei—both employing the full sun and moon block. There are, of course, differences, suggesting that each is exploring variations of the same theme.

If we look at them as *inside* entry techniques, however, it seems to suggest that the turns in the pattern of kata do not necessarily reinforce the martial principle of stepping off line or, put more colloquially, getting out of the way, that we see in other kata or even other styles of karate. (By way of comparison, it is important to remember here that the mawashi uke employed as an entry technique for each of the finishing techniques in the first half of Suparinpei moves initially to the *outside* of the opponent's attack.) While this principle does seem to hold true in the stepping patterns or techniques of *some* of the classical kata of Goju-ryu, it doesn't seem to be universal. Suparinpei kata, because the entry techniques move to the inside of the opponent's defensive posture, suggests that most of the turns, at least in the second half of the kata where we see complete sequences, merely signal the beginning of a new sequence.

In any case, the second and third steps of this sequence, moving forward in Basic Stance, are the same as what we see in the first complete sequence of Seisan kata. As the right foot steps forward, the right hand is brought up, palm first, stopping at shoulder level with the arm bent at the elbow. The angle of the arm is reminiscent of the arm position we see in the opening kamae of Sanchin kata, a position we often use as a reference point.

As the right step finishes, the right hand turns over—I am referring here to the usual timing we see in the performance of kata, not in how this technique is applied—in what appears to be the simulation of a grab. There are subtle differences shown in the final hand position as it is executed by different Goju schools. Some schools show the hand vertical with the palm facing forward, while other schools will show the palm down with the fingers pointing out to the side, similar to the open-hand chest block we see in the Gekisai kata. The differences, however, may be insignificant as long as the intention is clear, and the intention here is that the right hand is brought up to attack the opponent's neck with a *shuto uchi* (knife hand strike) and then control the head as the hand turns over.

The real problem we are faced with in the interpretation of kata, especially when we encounter these apparent differences—this instance being a prime example—is the rhythm that has crept into the performance of kata, influencing not only how we execute these movements but how we interpret them as well. This second sequence exhibits this sort of static posturing, where each of the movements seems to be given a separate time signature, as if it were disconnected from the rest of the body and the speed at which the sequential movements would need to be executed in application. That is: The right foot steps forward. Then the right arm is brought up and the left arm is brought down. Then the right hand is turned over. Then the left foot steps forward. Then the left arm is brought up and the right arm is brought down. Then the left hand is turned over. The movement looks robotic, the way we might first learn a kata.

This sort of tempo, however, with its disconnected movements, would never work in application. In order to "see" the bunkai in a series of dynamic movements like the second sequence of Suparinpei, we need to practice the fluid movement from the upward or rising open-hand strike or shuto to the controlling downward "block" done with the same arm. This is a complex movement and isn't easily captured in the juxtaposition of still photographs that one might find in a martial arts manual.

In this second sequence, as the right hand is brought up to attack the head or neck, the left hand is brought down, ending with the wrist bent and the palm facing down. The left hand is used to grab the opponent's right arm, pulling down, after the initial left semicircular rising block. The right shuto uchi to the side of the opponent's neck is the initial attack, but the right hand rotates almost immediately, beginning its downward

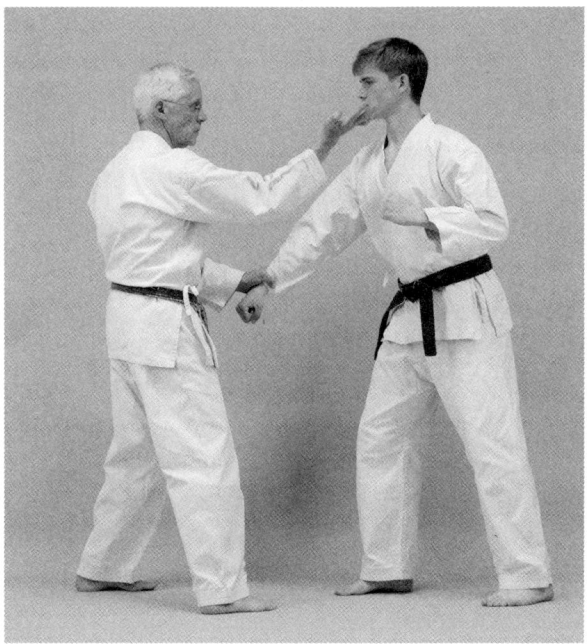

FIGURE 2.52 After the initial inside move, the defender steps in, grabbing the opponent's right arm and attacking the neck with the right-hand shuto.

semicircular motion, pulling down on the opponent's head as the defender steps forward into the next technique. In other words, the motion of the arms does not stop in order to rotate the hands.

This next step, into a left-foot-forward Basic Stance, is again the same as the left-foot-forward step we see in the first sequence of Seisan, and the technique functions the same way. As the left foot steps forward, the right hand is brought down into what looks like an open-hand lower-level block, and the left hand is brought up, palm first, stopping at shoulder level with the arm bent at the elbow. As we see in the performance of the kata, the left hand turns over as the step finishes, again simulating a grab of some kind or controlling technique.

As a point of comparison, we should note that in the old-school performance of these palm-up and palm-down techniques in the first sequence of Seisan kata, whether this technique is shown two times or four times, the last palm-up attack with the left hand does not turn over, but rather is brought in toward the chest before the pivot to the west and the continuation of the sequence. This is an important distinction to remember when considering the application of the final palm-up technique in the second sequence of Suparinpei and what the rotation of the palm implies.

The rotation of the hands that we see in the upper position of this technique is actually connected to the pulling down or lowering of the arm. Furthermore, the actual application of the technique against the opponent occurs somewhere in the middle of the two techniques—that is, in the space between the right hand being brought down and the left hand being brought up. The completed technique that we see in the performance of kata—with the left palm up at shoulder level and the right palm down at hip level—is the follow-through.

If we were to use an analogy, we might look at a golfer's swing. The golfer makes contact with the ball halfway through the 360 degrees of his or her golf swing. A baseball pitcher's arm finishes somewhere near the knee, but the release point is a good deal earlier. We don't look to explain what the pitcher's hand is doing in the still photograph that shows its proximity to the knee. Neither should we look to explain these techniques in the second sequence of Suparinpei by looking solely at the position of the hands at the completion of each technique.

The first, second, and third steps after the turn around in this second sequence from Suparinpei—that is, the step with the right, the step with the left, and again the step with the right—look the same, though they alternate sides. Some schools will do two additional steps, using the same techniques, just as two additional steps are often added to the first sequence of Seisan kata. What this indicates structurally about the kata, I believe, is that three of these techniques are meant to function together (two in the case of Seisan kata). The classical kata of Goju-ryu do not show needless repetition of techniques unless they are showing both a right and left side, which is what is probably indicated by the series of five of these techniques in some versions of Suparinpei.

It is certainly possible that there may be an alternate interpretation of these rising and downward palm techniques. In this version of the sequence, where we see three of these techniques—two with the right

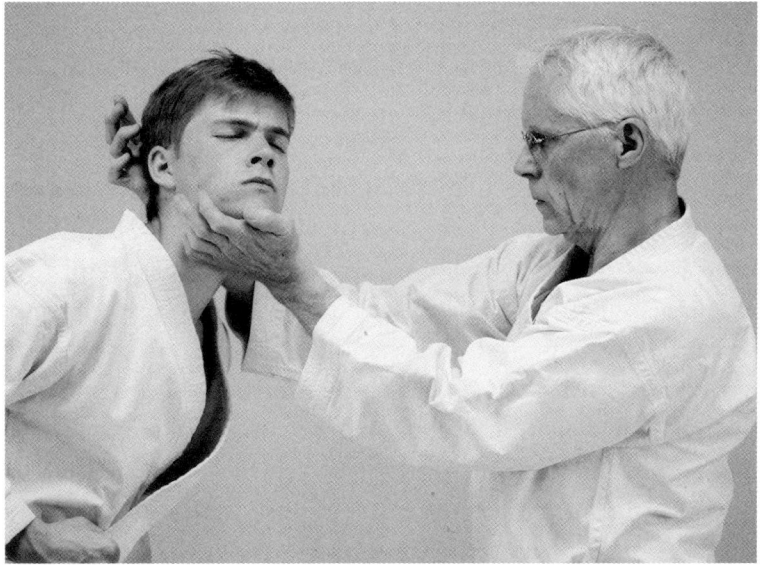

FIGURE 2.53 As the right hand begins to bring the attacker's head down, the left palm comes up to attack and control.

hand rising and one with the left—the message of the kata may simply be that only one of these techniques is used to precede the turning crescent kick or the jumping kick that follows it. In other words, the second of these techniques, done with the left rising palm, may simply be showing the technique on the other side—in other words, if the initial entry blocks were done with the opposite hands. In this case, the third technique, repeating the first rising palm strike, would be used simply to continue the sequence so that the finishing technique could be shown attached to the correct entry and controlling techniques. There are certainly other examples of this structure in the classical kata. In the first sequence of Seiunchin kata, for instance, the entry technique is shown three times—twice with a right-foot-forward shiko dachi and once with a left-foot-forward shiko dachi—before the finishing techniques are shown, tacked onto the third repetition.

Once again, one should remember that this step-by-step description of kata movement is, of course, how we learn kata, focusing on each individual movement. In application, however, there is much less distinction between each movement or technique. As the left foot steps forward into a left-foot-forward Basic Stance, the right hand has already begun to move downward and the left hand has already begun to move upward.

The left-foot-forward step, with the raising of the left palm, is where the left hand is brought up to attack and control the opponent's head. In fact, if one had control of the opponent's head here with the right hand, then this left hand technique might be used to twist the attacker's head by coming up into the attacker's chin and pushing out (fig. 2.53).

In one sense, since two palm-up techniques, coupled with the initial right and left circular blocks, seems to be enough to "finish" the opponent, it is difficult to say definitively whether the second and third palm-up techniques are both finishes, just showing the opposite side, or whether they are showing a continuation of the same side. In other words, the third of these palm-up techniques might be viewed merely as the finish technique of this sequence if it had begun on the opposite side—that is, if the kata had chosen to show these techniques beginning with a *left* circular down block and a *right* circular rising block. There is some justification for this view. We see a number of different instances of this structure in other classical kata where a sequence is shown on both the left and right sides, but the finishing technique is only shown on one side, attached to the second repetition. However, this sort of structure doesn't seem to apply to any other sequence of Suparinpei kata. What we also see fairly often in the classical subjects of Goju is that the opponent's head is first twisted in one direction and then quickly twisted back in the opposite direction. In the case of this second sequence of Suparinpei, this would suggest that the left rising open-hand technique might be used to push out, twisting the opponent's head in one direction, and then the third rising palm, the right hand, is brought up to twist the opponent's head in the opposite direction.

When we see these same techniques in Seisan kata, after the same initial entry technique, the right shuto uchi comes in to attack the neck as the right foot steps forward. Then, stepping forward with the left foot, the left hand is brought up, and, pushing in on the opponent's chin, the defender pivots to the right (west), twisting the opponent's head—the head is first twisted in and then forcefully snapped back in the other direction. One of the obvious differences in Seisan, however, is that the hands close, indicating that one hand is grabbing the hair or topknot and the other is wrapped around the opponent's chin. We see a picture of this in one of the sketches associated with the *Bubishi* (fig. 2.54), what has been referred to as the Bible of Okinawan karate.

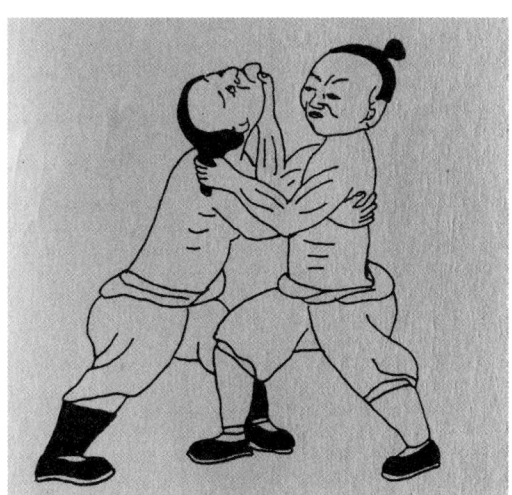

FIGURE 2.54 This line drawing from the *Bubishi* depicts a head-twisting technique that we see in Seisan kata and in Suparinpei kata.

It is difficult to determine or to state categorically where the actual finishing technique is in this sequence. The number of steps alone introduces a certain degree of ambiguity. Does the sequence finish with the rising left hand attack, twisting the head, or does it require an additional step, finishing with the second rising right hand attack? In Seisan kata, which seems to show a variation of these same techniques in its first sequence, the finishing head twist occurs with the pivot to the right, or west, into a right-foot-forward Basic Stance. This would seem to support the idea that we need the third of these rising palm attacks in Suparinpei for the finishing neck break. In most instances in the classical subjects, the opponent's head is first twisted in one direction and then twisted back in the opposite direction.

Another possibility one should consider is that each of the rising palm attacks introduces one of the two alternative finishing techniques that immediately follows: the turning crescent kick alternative and the jumping kick and elbow attack alternative; the right rising palm position beginning the turn into the crescent kick, and the left rising palm position illustrating the position from which the jumping kick is initiated.

Yet another possibility, although it doesn't fundamentally change the bunkai, is that the hands may change moving from the left rising palm attack to the last right rising palm attack. After the left rising palm attack, the left hand could just as easily be used to control the opponent's head—depending, of course, on how the opponent moved in response to the previous technique—and the right hand could be brought up to the opponent's chin for the final head-twisting technique.

It is difficult to know because we only have the one side, kata, half the equation, to figure out what the whole picture would look like, to mix metaphors. The bunkai is fundamentally the same. Is the ambiguity intentional? Perhaps the kata is simply showing us different possibilities that may arise in any situation as dynamic and subject to change as a serious confrontation that may require one to use these kinds of techniques. We might also note here the similarity of these palm-up techniques to the final technique of Shisochin kata, suggesting that there, too, the palm techniques are used to twist the opponent's head, and in Saifa kata, just before the kicks.

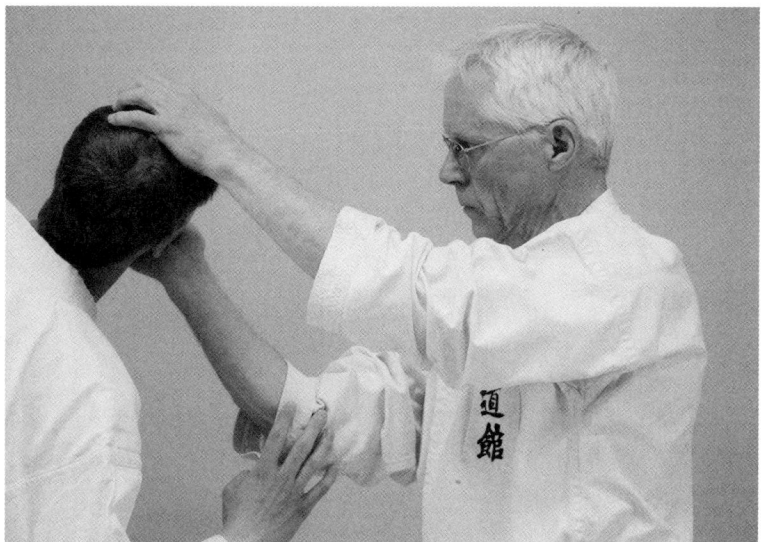

FIGURE 2.55 If a hand change is employed, the left hand is used to control the opponent's head as the right rising palm is brought up into the chin, twisting the head.

Again, anything is possible, but I'm not a big fan of any argument that employs the idea of intentional ambiguity. The strongest argument to me is that this sequence in Suparinpei seems to be a variation of the first sequence of Seisan kata (or vice versa). Where Seisan kata *pivots* to the right, into a right-foot-forward Basic Stance, twisting the attacker's head, Suparinpei steps *forward* into a right-foot-forward Basic Stance.[10]

The Turning Crescent Kick Alternative

See figures 3.49–51.

This series of techniques seems to begin with what appears to be a turn into a left palm-up middle-level block to the north or the original front of the kata. It is certainly one of the more problematic sequences of movements in Suparinpei. This is due in part to the turning or spinning crescent kick. Because it doesn't occur anywhere else in the classical canon of

Goju-ryu, there is no point of reference, no other instance that might help in determining how it is meant to be used here.

However, the middle-level block itself is also a bit of an enigma. Each of the complete sequences in Suparinpei begins with the same entry or receiving technique—one arm moving in a semicircular fashion with the palm or forearm pressing down, finishing in the gedan position, and the other arm moving up in a semicircular fashion with the palm facing forward. Structurally (and thematically), it doesn't seem in keeping with the general tenor of the kata that a new sequence would begin with a completely different entry technique.

If we were to imagine that this was an entry technique and meant to be employed in the same manner as the other entry techniques—against a two-armed attack or grappling posture from the opponent—then the right

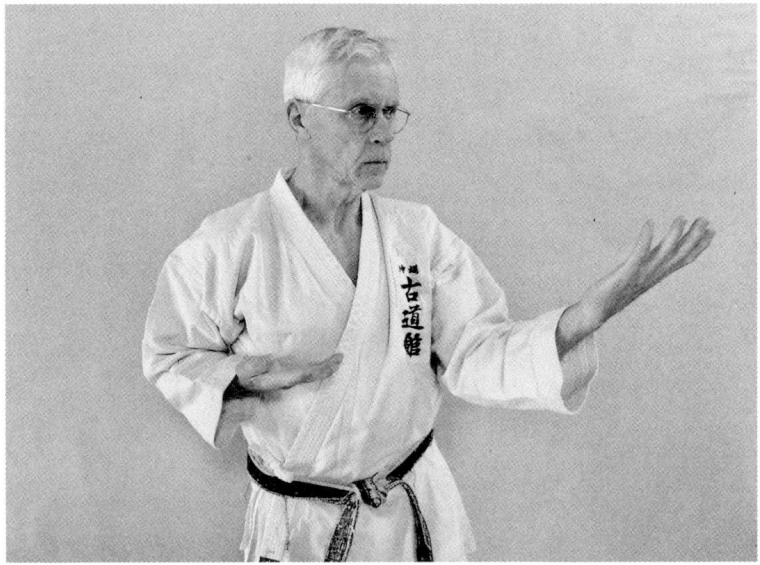

FIGURE 2.56 The final position of this technique, what we see reproduced in still photographs, shows the left hand, palm up, with the fingertips at shoulder level, with the right hand, palm up, held alongside the ribs. The angle of the bend in the left arm should again recall the kamae posture of Sanchin kata.

arm would be blocking the opponent's left arm, for example, and the left palm-up block would come inside the opponent's right arm. But it is still unclear exactly how the crescent kick would be used or what the target of the kick would be. In any event, it doesn't seem terribly lethal by itself, though there have been many options suggested.[11]

While kicking techniques do occur at the end of many sequences in the classical subjects, they are never the sole finishing technique, always occurring after a head-twisting technique of some kind. The position of the arms is also questionable, unless something has been left out. The defender's right arm does not seem to have control of the attacker's left arm in quite the same way as we see in the other entry techniques, and, since the left hand is palm-up, of course, this is probably true of the defender's left arm as well. All in all, it doesn't seem to be an effective entry technique.

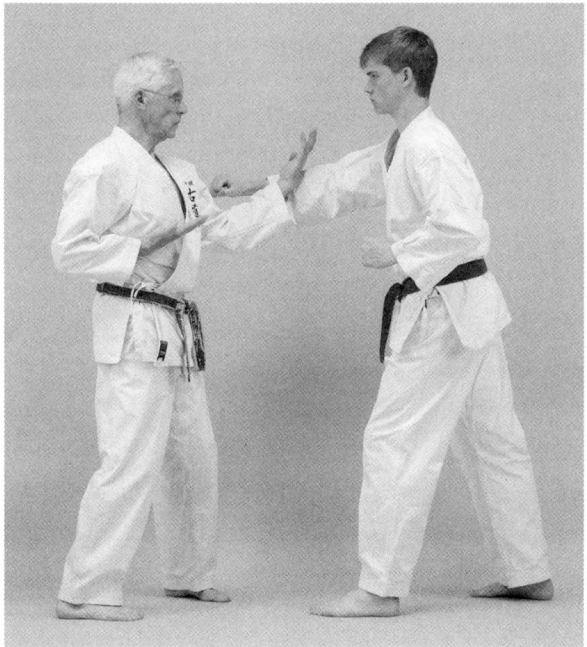

FIGURE 2.57 Using the left palm-up block in a similar fashion as the other entry techniques in Suparinpei kata.

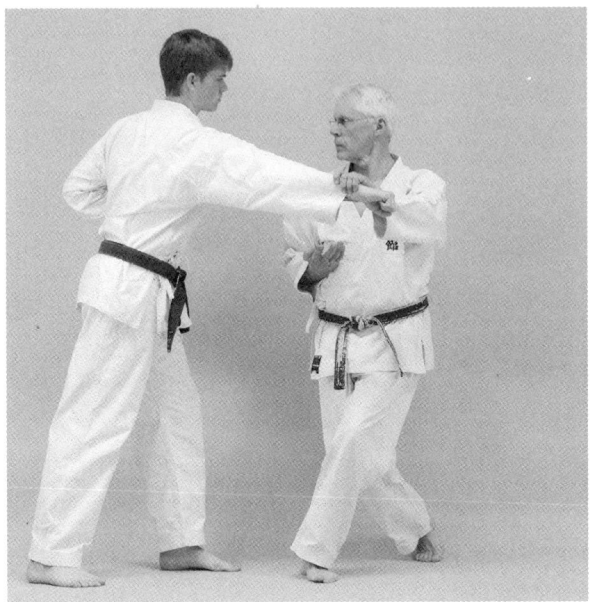

FIGURE 2.58 Using the left palm-up block in this
way helps to pull the opponent off balance but leaves
the defender open to the opponent's attack with the
other hand.

I would suggest, therefore, that the more probable explanation—though
the reasoning behind this idiosyncratic and seemingly illogical structure is
hard to rationalize—is that this middle-level palm-up block is meant to be
seen as a continuation of the previous sequence; that like the first complete
sequence in Seisan kata, which it closely resembles, this second sequence of
Suparinpei is meant to finish with a kicking technique, even though the last
of the south-facing palm-up techniques suggests a head-twisting neck break
that would probably in itself be a sufficient finishing technique.

However, there is still a question of exactly how the middle-level
palm-up "block" to the north is meant to be connected to the second
sequence. The most likely method is that the defender would bring the
inside of the left forearm up into the opponent's neck on the turn to the
front, after the last of the palm-up attacks.

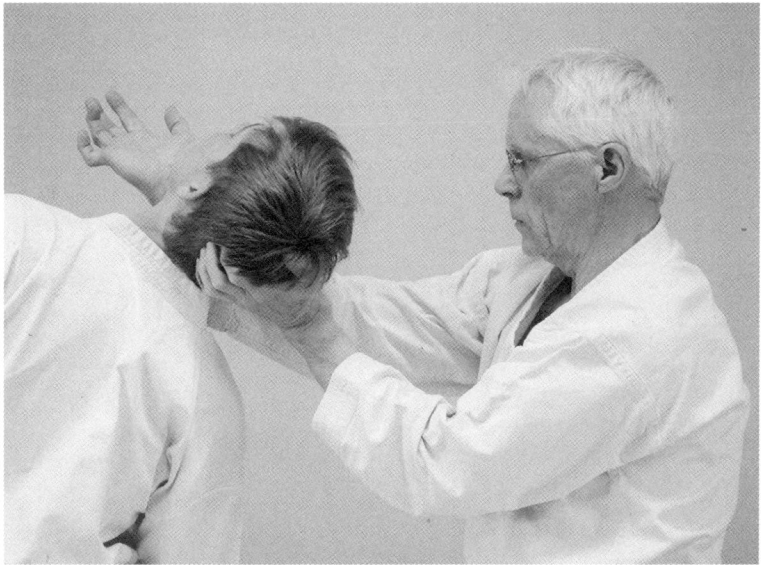

FIGURE 2.59 Beginning from the right palm-up attack—the second or the fourth technique in this sequence—the right hand carries the head around to the original front (north) of the kata, as the defender pivots in a counterclockwise direction.

After this last head attack—with the defender's left hand on the head and the right hand on the opponent's chin—the defender's right hand or forearm pushes on the attacker's head, pushing to the left, counterclockwise, toward the original front of the kata. As the defender executes this turn, the left forearm is brought up into the opponent's neck (fig. 2.60). The defender's hands have effectively changed at this point. This is the position we see when this technique is broken down into still photographs—facing the original front of the kata in a left-foot-forward Basic Stance with the left palm up in what appears to be a middle-level block (fig. 3.49). One should remember, however, that the techniques of a given sequence should be continuous, without any gaps or pauses in their execution.

In continuing to turn in a counterclockwise direction, the defender's left hand and forearm rotate, bringing the attacker's head down in order

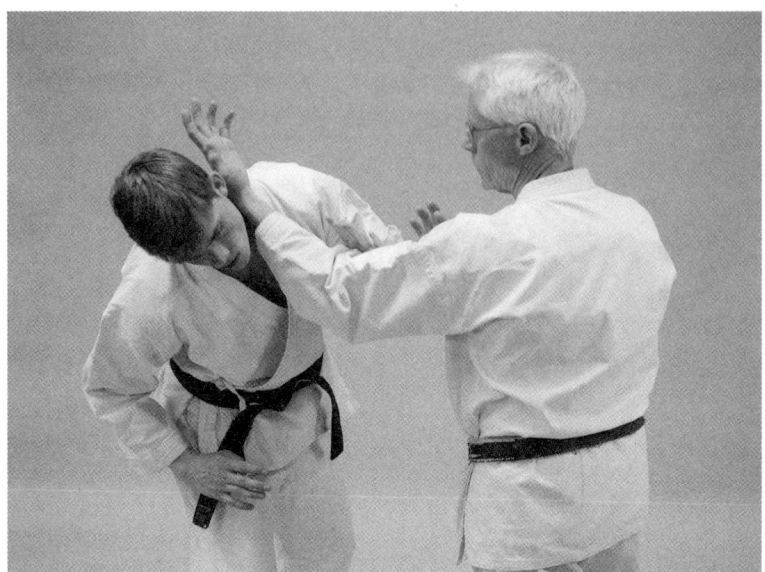

FIGURE 2.60 Using the palm-up forearm block, in conjunction with the previous technique, begins to unbalance the opponent and bring the head down. However, it is important to remember that the technique does not stop here. This is a forearm controlling technique that occurs repeatedly in Kururunfa kata. It is most apparent as the first technique of the third sequence in Kururunfa, though even there it is meant to be attached to the opening entry technique of the kata.

· to finish with the crescent kick (fig. 2.61), using the shin to attack the opponent's neck. The 180-degree counterclockwise turn to the original front, in this case, does not signal the beginning of a new sequence, only an alternative ending to the second sequence. The turn is necessary to pull the opponent off balance, bringing the head down for the crescent kick attack. This somewhat unusual use of the inside forearm technique is similar to the use of the forearm in the second circular block in the last sequence of Suparinpei kata. Both use the defender's left forearm against the left side of the attacker's neck to bring the head down.

This inside forearm technique, where the defender's left forearm is brought up to attack the left side of the opponent's neck, for example,

can be seen repeatedly in Kururunfa kata. It acts as a transitioning control technique between the core position of the first sequence—where,
for example, the right arm, with elbow down and palm up, is held in a
Sanchin-like position to the front, and the left arm, with the palm down,
is held in what appears to be a lower blocking position or what is sometimes interpreted as a knife-edge attack to the opponent's lower abdo-
men—and each of the subsequent sequences. That is, the second, third,
and fourth sequences of the kata are shown without this initial entry
technique. This accounts for the unique structure of Kururunfa kata, and
in particular the three palm-up and palm-down techniques that follow
the opening left and right side kicking techniques. The connection to
this second sequence of Suparinpei is most apparent in moving from this
palm-up and palm-down technique into the third sequence of Kururunfa
where, again, we see the same palm-up middle-level "block" in Basic
Stance that we see in this sequence of Suparinpei, and they should both
be applied in the same way.

Though this is, no doubt, the more likely application of the palm-up
middle-level block and crescent kick, there is another possible way to
employ this technique. For this application, coming off the last palm-up
attack of the second sequence (facing south)—with again the defender's
left hand holding the opponent's head or hair and the right hand having
twisted the chin—the defender would turn counterclockwise 180 degrees
to the north, pulling the opponent forward and off balance with the left
hand, bringing the opponent's head down.

This use of the forearm "block," though here it is executed in Basic
Stance, should remind us of the forearm "blocking" technique in shiko
dachi that we see in the first half of Suparinpei kata (fig. 2.33), where it
is executed to the four corners or ordinal directions. There it is shown
as a bridging or controlling technique attached to the initial mawashi
uke. I would argue the same case with this palm-up middle-level block
in Basic Stance. It is not meant to be an initial entry technique, no matter
which way it is applied. It and the jumping kick series that follows are
alternative endings to the second sequence of the kata.

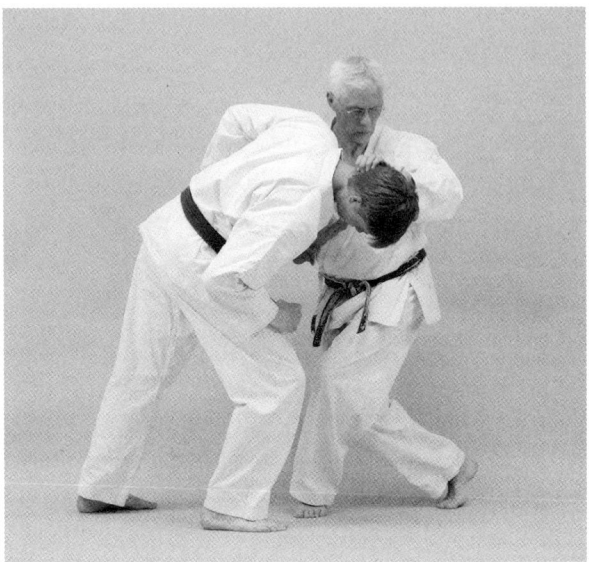

FIGURE 2.61 The left palm-up technique continues
with a counterclockwise rotation, controlling the opponent's head with the left arm, prior to the crescent kick.

It is probably worth repeating that to see the real effect of this on the
opponent, it is important to remember that the technique does not stop
at that artificial end point, standing in a left-foot-forward Basic Stance,
facing north, with the left arm palm-up—what we see represented in the
illustrations of martial arts manuals, including this one. We may need to
teach this way, as it makes instruction, particularly of large groups, easier,
and certainly it is easier to learn if we break complicated movements up
into smaller pieces, but the technique continues through this point to the
execution of the spinning crescent kick.

The timing may be the greatest impediment in being able to "see"
the application of this technique, or, indeed, many of the techniques
we see in the classical subjects of Goju. When we perform any of these
movements in kata, we generally do so with a good deal of deliberation,
often punctuating a sequence more for the performance than to display an understanding of how the techniques are used. And sadly, our

understanding of a kata is often judged on the aesthetics of the performance. It all creates a situation that is more confusing than enlightening.

There may often be a number of plausible explanations for how a given technique in kata may be applied, some better than others. For the most part, I believe, they all center on how we should best understand the structure of the kata—that is, what is the message implied in how the different techniques are put together in a single kata. This order is certainly not arbitrary. Hopefully, as with the above examples, the general idea is usually the same, or at least quite similar, following along the same thematic understanding of the kata. That means that any explanation should fit the structure of the kata, follow its general tenor or themes, and conform to sound martial principles. One of those principles in the classical kata of Goju-ryu is that the defender should have control of the opponent before kicking or using the legs. This is one of the principles that raises the issue of how we should understand the techniques of the second sequence and the series of moves that follow it—the series of techniques that includes the palm-up block and crescent kick and the jumping kick series of moves.

The Jumping Kick and Elbow Attack Alternative

See figures 3.52–56.
With this next series of techniques, we are again facing the original front of the kata. The kata finishes the crescent kick and turn in a left-foot-forward Basic Stance in what seems to be the open-hand blocking position, or at least a close approximation of it. This is followed by a jumping kick, pushing off with the right rear leg and elevating with the left forward leg, and then kicking with the right leg, landing in a right-foot-forward Horse Stance. The right elbow is then brought into the left palm—the same technique that we see in the first sequence of Suparinpei after the front kick (fig. 3.39). The right arm then unfolds, again identical in appearance to the first sequence, with the right forearm vertical and the left hand held along

the inside of the right forearm. Unlike the first sequence, however, this sequence usually finishes here, with what some imagine to be a supported back-fist strike or uraken, a technique that is hardly lethal and hardly in keeping with the tenor of the kata.

Certainly it does not appear that this sequence is connected to the previous crescent kick sequence, and since there is a directional change, it is tempting to consider that these techniques constitute a sequence of their own. However, there is something that feels just a bit unrealistic about following this initial open-hand position—since neither hand seems to be a blocking or receiving technique—with a jumping kick. There is an old saying that one should kick only when one has at least three feet on the ground. The message, of course, is that one should kick only when one is well grounded, balanced, and has hold of the opponent, therefore utilizing at least one of the defender's legs and both of the opponent's legs for balance and stability, while ensuring that the opponent cannot destroy one's own balance. It would be questionable to initiate any attack with a kick unless one were already in control of the opponent. And in that case, we would have to ask how the defender got control of the opponent. The hand position we see in the kata, after the completion of the crescent kick and turn back to the front, doesn't seem as though it is initiating a blocking or controlling technique. Any kick in this situation would merely push the opponent away.

Even if we choose to ignore the issue of an inadequate controlling technique, however, there is the question of why one would use a jumping kick at all when the rear-leg front kick we see in the first sequence seems to be the logical way to bring the opponent's head down in order to attack with the same right elbow technique. And the only scenario that seems to provide an answer, I think, is that this series of techniques, like the one before it, is structurally meant to be attached to the end of the second sequence, whether that is the left palm-up shuto attack, the right palm-up shuto attack, or the left palm-up, inside forearm "block"—in other words, it is not clear structurally exactly where, in the previous sequence of moves, one should attach the jumping kick.

We see this sort of fragmented structure at the beginning of Suparinpei, where the mawashi uke and nukite/shuto act as the initial receiving or entry

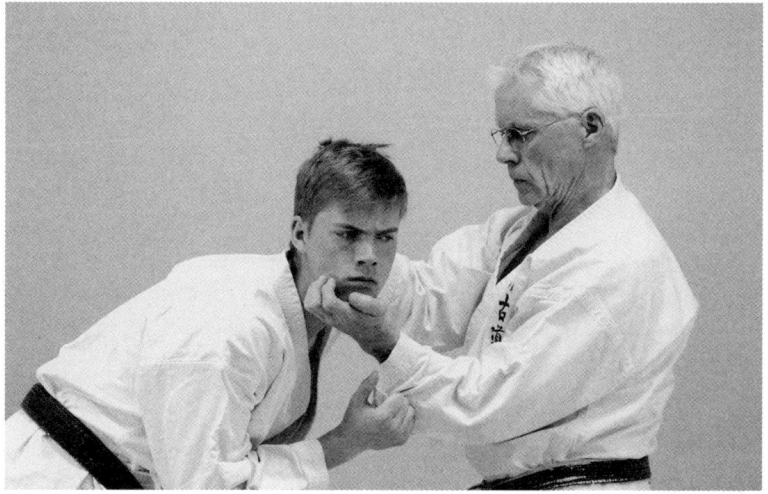

FIGURE 2.62 The double jumping kick series begins here, attached to this technique of the second complete sequence. One should remember, however, that the movement is dynamic; the left hand is on the way up as the right hand is being brought down.

techniques for the three series of techniques that follow it—the mawashi in Cat Stance, the double "punch," and the shiko dachi angle techniques. The complete mawashi uke and nukite/shuto technique we see at the beginning of Suparinpei, though only shown on one side, shows one hand on the top or the back of the opponent's head with the other hand on the chin—the same position one sees in the earlier illustration from the *Bubishi*.

It is also similar to the position of the hands toward the end of the second complete sequence, in this case, the next-to-last step to the south before the kata shows a turn into the left palm-up forearm technique that initiates the crescent kick (see fig. 2.53), or, in fact, if the hand change is employed, the last step in the sequence (see fig. 2.55).

From this position, with the opponent's head held relatively high, it makes sense to jump in order to attack the head with one or both knees, landing squarely in a stable Horse Stance as the opponent is brought down. I can imagine that the left knee is merely used for elevation while the right knee is used as the primary attack to the opponent's head, or the left knee being brought up to attack the head as the right foot follows with a kick to the opponent's body. The right elbow is then brought into the left palm, which, in application, has more to do with the twisting of the opponent's head than attacking with the elbow, as the defender would already be grasping the head. At this point, similar to what we see in the first sequence of the kata, the right arm is "unfolded" until the forearm is vertical, as the left hand maintains contact with the right forearm. This is the head twist. (Curiously, this unfolding into a vertical forearm technique is very similar to the technique we see at the end of the second sequence in Seipai kata, and, I would argue, they are meant to function in a similar way.)

Since much of this sequence looks identical to the movements of the first sequence, it is tempting to interpret them in the same manner—that is, it is natural to assume that techniques that appear the same must be doing the same thing. This is not always the case, however, as we see over and over again in a number of other classical kata. And, I would argue, it is not the case here either, particularly since the sequence usually ends here, with the unfolding of the right arm and vertical positioning of the right forearm, not showing the same final head-twisting technique we see in the first sequence. Some have even gone so far as to assume that some techniques have been purposely left out of kata to hide the actual applications. This seems to me a weak and self-serving notion, feeding our natural desires to perpetuate these myths of secrecy and giving some the license to dismiss any stumbling blocks they encounter in the analysis of kata with the ready reply that they are merely filling in the gaps.

Yet thematically, if we see this series of techniques as a continuation of the second of the circular palm-up techniques of the second sequence, with its right-hand head grab and left shuto or nukite, then the final twisting of the opponent's head is simply accomplished in a slightly different way. It is unclear whether this jumping technique and elbow attack would be attached to the second or third of these semicircular palm-up techniques to the south. It is certainly possible to accomplish the final head-twisting technique from the third of these semicircular palm-up techniques—that is, if the head or hair is in the left hand and the right hand is on the chin. The hands in the second position, however, seems preferable. In fact, one would be tempted to argue that this second sequence of Suparinpei, for whatever reason, seems as though it may be showing three possible finishing techniques: the first of these being the third of the right palm-up techniques used to twist the opponent's neck as the left hand holds the attacker's hair; the second being the use of the crescent kick; and the third being the jumping kick and "elbow" technique.

The sequence, in other words, shows a variation. And though it may certainly be gruesome, and not something we would want to test out on a training partner, it is not difficult to imagine what happens in this scenario after the jumping kick.

As the defender lands in Horse Stance, the right hand, which has hold of the attacker's hair, is brought in, toward the chest, while the left hand, which has hold of the attacker's chin, is pushed forward, twisting the opponent's head in one direction. Then, the right arm is "unfolded" until the forearm is vertical, pulling up on the opponent's hair, as the left hand, which has hold of the attacker's chin, pulls in until the hand is brought into position along the inside of the right forearm. The effect of this technique is to twist the attacker's head and break the neck. The first

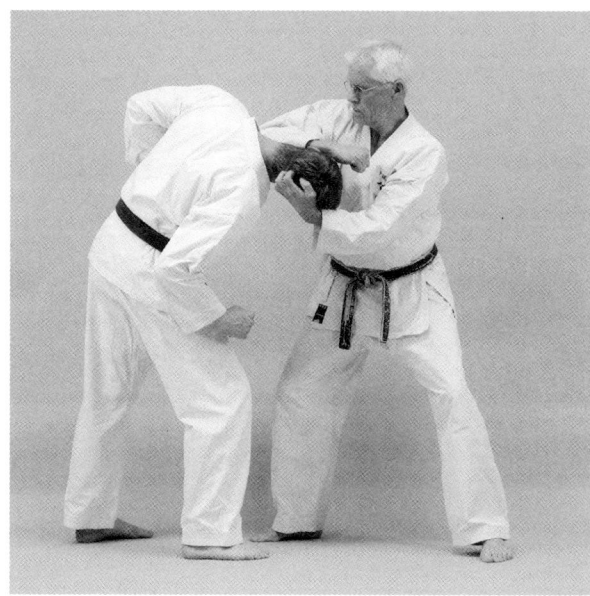

FIGURE 2.63 We often look at this as an elbow attack, but it may be more instructive to focus on the right and left hands in this case.

twisting motion, pulling down and in, is on a more or less horizontal plane, while the second twisting motion pushes in and out on a different plane—very similar to the twisting motion we see in the semicircular palm-up and palm-down techniques of the second sequence of the kata.

I have on occasion had students tell me that these descriptions are difficult to "see." Perhaps that's one of the lamentable effects of so much "oyo" bunkai—though I am hesitant to use the term—that one encounters on the internet and elsewhere. I had never heard the term *oyo bunkai* in Okinawa or in training with my teacher, Kimo Wall sensei. In one sense, it seems to me, "oyo bunkai" has come to stand for any creative interpretation of kata technique, regardless of whether or not it adheres to the movements one performs in solo kata. I think this "anything goes" attitude is regrettable and really makes kata analysis more confusing than it needs to be. I think descriptions of bunkai, whether they are accompanied by pictures or not, are relatively easy to "see" if we stick strictly to the movements we see in kata. I have often told students to "just do the kata," when they seem to struggle with applying a technique against a training partner.

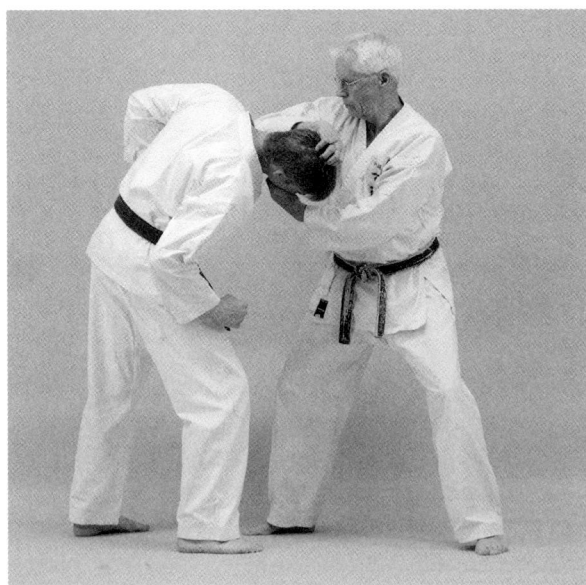

FIGURE 2.64 When the right arm is "unfolded," the attacker's head and chin are pulled back with a twisting motion.

The Last Sequence

See figures 3.57–60.

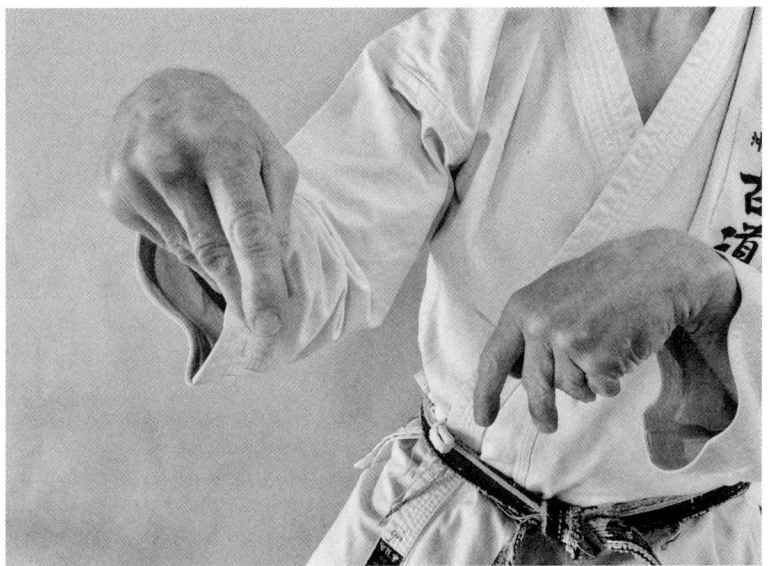

FIGURE 2.65 The position of the hands in the last posture of the kata
is the result of the technique applied between this posture and the previous spear hand.

The last sequence of Suparinpei kata is really very simple, as it borrows techniques from both Seisan kata and Sanseiru kata. The crux of this sequence,
one might say, is what appears to be a right spear-hand thrust in shiko dachi
with the left open hand brought in toward the shoulder (see fig. 3.59).
As has so often been said, however, appearances can be deceiving.

Language can also be deceiving. If we call it a spear-hand thrust, we
begin to assume—particularly because most of these techniques are done
with a certain amount of explosive force in the demonstration of kata—
that this is an attack executed with the tips of the extended fingers. This
alone often prompts students to train with all manner of apparatus to
strengthen the fingers for just this kind of attack. We might see students

strike the makiwara repeatedly with the fingertips. Or we might see them standing over a bucket filled with sand or pebbles, thrusting their hands in until the tips of their fingers are numb.

Our expectations play a significant role here as well. For most, karate has come to be characterized by punches and kicks or, more broadly, percussive attacks, whether those attacks are with the fist, the foot, the wrist, or a spear hand. We generally see what we expect to see. In other words, *how* we train tends to inform the way that we analyze kata. It's difficult to step back and look at things, in Shunryu Suzuki's words, with a "beginner's mind."

What should really inform our analysis, however, are the techniques that we see in the previous sequences of the kata—because the classical subjects are generally organized around various themes—and how we see some of these same techniques employed in other kata, particularly Seisan and Sanseiru in this case.

The first technique of the last sequence is actually a more complete expression of the sun and moon block that we see in the Shodokan (Higa) version of Seisan kata. After the final technique of the previous sequence— the "unfolding," head-twisting technique in shiko dachi we see in "The Jumping Kick and Elbow Attack Alternative," above—Suparinpei again shows a counterclockwise turn to the left to face the south. This is the same turn we see in the second sequence, and once again we are using the right downward semicircular blocking motion and the left rising semicircular blocking motion to move inside the opponent's two-arm clinch or grappling posture (and, of course, the technique is equally applicable against two punches, as has been said).

This initial two-handed technique is immediately followed by what appears to be another two-handed circular blocking motion—both arms moving in the same counterclockwise direction but at slightly offset intervals—while at the same time shifting or sliding forward into a left-foot-forward Horse Stance. This is followed by the right spear-hand thrust with the left palm being brought in toward the right shoulder. Then, stepping around to face the original front of the kata (north), the hands circle, as if holding a small ball, ending in the familiar double "crane's beak" or "dog" posture in shiko dachi that has come to characterize Suparinpei kata—a particularly graceful and enigmatic-looking posture.

This last sequence, and particularly the movements that lead up to and include this last posture, seems to present a difficult challenge to the imagination for most, perhaps even a test of one's understanding of Goju-ryu. It cannot really be taken apart, as is so often done, and applied piecemeal. That is, one should be careful not to treat finishing positions— this is one example—as if they were self-contained or were meant to include a receiving and an attacking technique in themselves. In some interpretations of this position, practitioners have imagined that the left hand is used to block and hook the opponent's arm, while the right hand is brought up to attack the head or neck with either the top of the bent wrist or the downward-pointing fingertips. There is a lot wrong with this interpretation.

Neither can the stances, steps, or directional changes be ignored. All of the pieces must fit together. Ultimately, this is one of the tests of any interpretation, theory, or analysis of kata. That is: Can we find an explanation that includes every aspect of a particular series of movements? And, of course, it must also be logical, realistic, and end the confrontation.

The initial receiving technique is once again the sun and moon block— itself a technique very much akin to the ubiquitous mawashi uke—with a turn into a left-foot-forward Basic Stance. The right arm is brought across and down in a counterclockwise semicircular fashion with the palm or forearm pressing down and finishing in the gedan position. The left arm follows, moving up and out in a counterclockwise semicircular fashion with the palm facing forward (fig. 2.66).

Using the complete sun and moon block (which, of course, includes the second of the circular arm motions), the defender's left hand grabs and pulls down and in on the attacker's right arm to control and unbalance the opponent, while the defender's right open hand is brought up to attack the opponent's head or face (fig. 2.67).

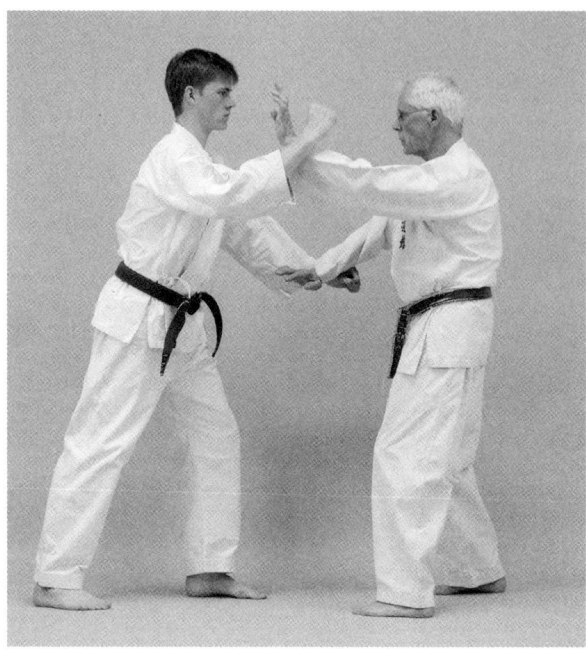

FIGURE 2.66 The first of the circular arm movements of the sun and moon block brings the defender inside the opponent's defenses or on the inside of both arms.

The vertical palm strike or *shotei tsuki* seen here in Suparinpei—rather than the straight punch *(choku tsuki)* or reverse punch *(gyaku tsuki)* practiced with such dogged persistence on the makiwara in traditional dojo and routinely employed as the finishing technique in yakusoku kumite drills—is the dominant *percussive* hand technique in the Kaishu kata of Goju. If the focus of one's training is on the classical kata, then one's solo practice should probably focus on developing one's palm (which might include the shuto or knife-edge attack) and forearm strikes rather than what seems to be the more conventional closed-hand striking that seems to be the primary focus not only of makiwara training but also of basic drills in many dojo. This is not to suggest that a strong punch is not an effective tool to have in one's arsenal of self-defense, only that the classical or koryu kata of Goju-ryu do not seem to emphasize the straight punch at all, ironic as that may seem for a technique that has, for many at least, come to characterize modern karate.

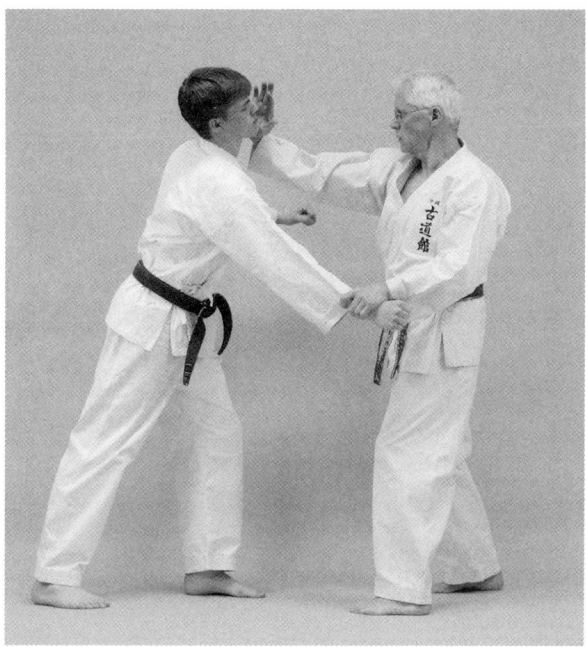

FIGURE 2.67 Using the start of the second circle of the sun and moon block, the opponent is pulled off balance and attacked with the right palm strike.

The next technique, a shift forward into a left-foot-forward shiko dachi or Horse Stance, serves to unbalance the attacker while moving in to control the opponent's head. From the previous palm strike, the defender's left arm is brought up under the right, moving in a counter-clockwise semicircular fashion, contacting the left side of the opponent's neck and pushing down or out as the defender shifts forward into Horse Stance (fig. 2.68).

It may be of interest to note that this use of the sun and moon block coupled with a shift forward into shiko dachi can also be found in the second sequence of Seisan kata. In fact, the beginning of this last sequence in Suparinpei and the second sequence of Seisan are quite similar, differing only after the execution of the sun and moon block. Where Suparinpei shows what seems to be a spear-hand thrust, Seisan shows what would seem to be three middle-level punches. What is of particular interest, however, given the similarity of the openings, is that Seisan is most likely illustrating a variation in the application of the sun and moon block. That is, the second sequence of Seisan kata shows us how to deal with an opponent that blocks the defender's right open-hand palm strike that we see in figure 2.67. If the opponent, using his or her left arm, continues to "stick" to the defender's right arm, deflecting the palm strike, then the defender simply continues with the rest of the sequence of moves we see in Seisan, bringing his or her left arm around, under the right arm, and grabbing the opponent's left arm, moving forward into the left-foot-forward shiko dachi.

The use of the Horse Stance to lower one's center of gravity and the use of the forward shifting movement in both Seisan and Suparinpei are important in order to bring the opponent's head down with this forearm technique, especially since the technique is being used in a predominantly straight line attack. In Suparinpei, the opponent's head is pushed down to the defender's left, allowing the defender the space to step around the opponent to execute the final head-twisting technique to the original front of the kata.

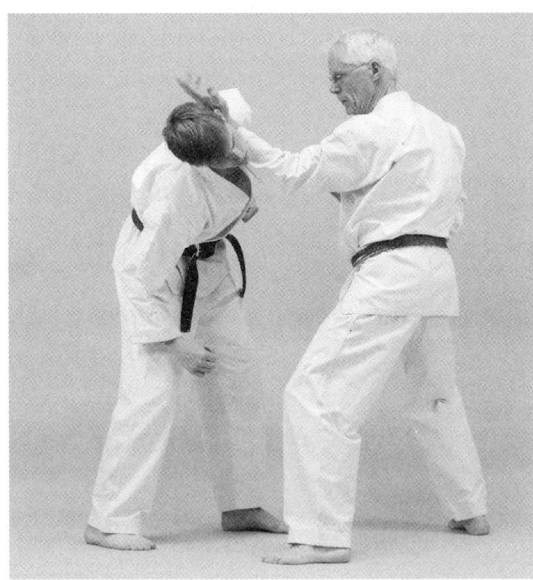

FIGURE 2.68 After the completion of the second circle of the sun and moon block, the opponent's head has been brought down. From this position of control, of course, the defender might counterattack with any number of techniques. The rest of the sequence shows one of these possibilities.

We see a similar use of this kind of forearm bridging or controlling technique being used in the second sequence in conjunction with the spinning crescent kick. In that case, the momentum of the turn, coupled with the pushing rotation of the forearm, is used to bring the opponent's head down for the finishing kick. In this last sequence, it is the use of the right palm strike and the shift or sliding stance, moving forward from a more upright Basic Stance into a lower Horse Stance, that serves to bring the opponent's head down. And, of course, the circular motion of the arms is continuous.

The next technique in this sequence of moves is the spear-hand thrust. This is probably a misnomer or at best merely describes the appearance of the technique. The purpose of the spear hand is to thrust the right arm under the opponent's neck. It doesn't need to be done with very much force or speed, unless one were to use the right forearm to attack the opponent's neck or throat. This is certainly a possibility. However, the primary intent, I believe, is to be able to control the top of the opponent's head with the left hand and place the right hand in a position to grab the opponent's chin.

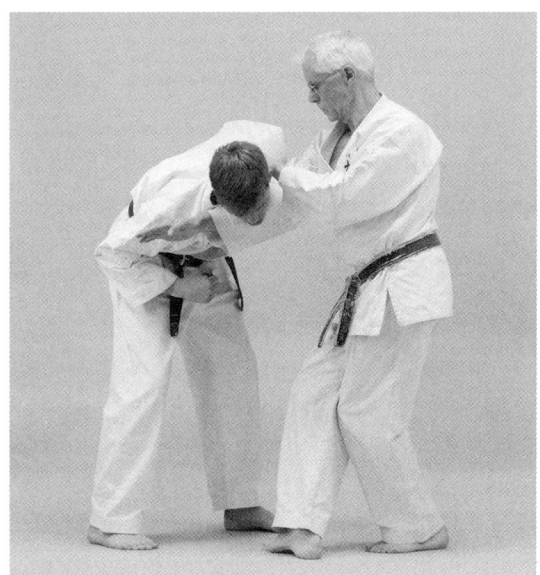

FIGURE 2.69 Although it is often referred to as a spear-hand attack, it is the forearm rather than the hand that may be used to attack the opponent's neck.

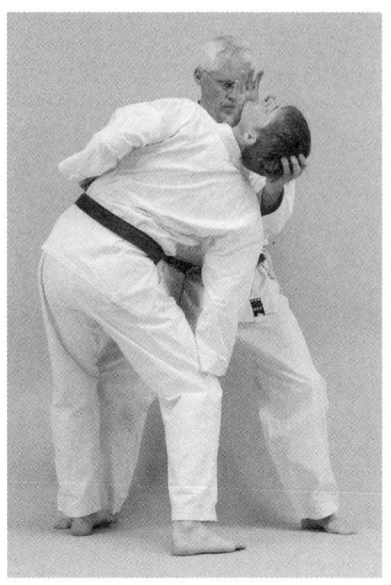

FIGURE 2.70 The purpose of the spear hand is to thrust the right arm under the opponent's chin. From that position, it is possible to grab the opponent's chin with the right hand and, turning to the original front, twist the head by pulling in and then pushing out and over with the right hand, while holding the head with the left hand.

The final technique in Suparinpei involves a turn to the original front (north) of the kata, while holding and twisting the opponent's head. Sometimes this is done by merely stepping across with the left foot and, facing the front, sinking into a right-foot-forward shiko dachi. Others will first take a short cross-step with the right foot before moving the left foot into a forward-facing shiko dachi. It really only depends on how much room we might need in order to manipulate the opponent. (It may be of interest to note that the differences one sees in the performance of kata often seem only to point to idiosyncratic preferences—that is, how different teachers or schools thought to accomplish the same bunkai. Whether one steps only with the left foot in this final technique from Suparinpei or uses a right cross-step prior to stepping with the left foot is one of these examples.)

There is also some variation in how the arms circle, and this, of course, is something that can't be adequately described with words, even if we add a series of still pictures. The simplest technique—one that can sometimes be seen in videos of older practitioners from previous generations—is done by merely turning to the front while holding the top of the opponent's head or hair with the left hand and pulling up on the opponent's chin with the right hand (fig. 2.71). This does not have the same flourish that one usually sees in the performance of Suparinpei kata, but in application it accomplishes the same thing.

There are a number of ways one might twist the opponent's head from the spear-hand position. Perhaps this accounts for the variety of ways we see this final technique demonstrated. The only guide we have, in this case, may be the imagination; it is difficult, and certainly not advisable, to practice this technique on a partner. But one should be able to watch the performance of the technique—and really this is true of any kata and any other technique—and "see" the bunkai, even if we are only seeing one side of it in a solo kata demonstration. Sadly, I find that there are many high-level performances that exhibit a good deal of athleticism and dramatic flair but very little understanding of the applications of the kata—you can't "see" the bunkai in the moves. It reminds me of something my teacher once said: that there might be a number of right ways to do something, but there are also many wrong ways. The hands work in opposition here, as they do in many of the finishing techniques of the classical kata. When we see a performance of kata where the practitioner demonstrates this final technique of Suparinpei, without showing this opposing movement of the hands, we might justifiably question his or her understanding of the kata.

It may be interesting to note here that the peculiar hand position—what has given the posture its various names, being reminiscent of a dog's paws or the beak of a bird—is really just a result of holding the head of the attacker and twisting it. If we are bent on trying to find exactly how the fingers should be held, or the angle the wrist should conform to, or how far away from the body each hand should be held at the completion of the kata, we are really missing the point. These things are important when we are looking at the proper execution of receiving or controlling techniques, at least to some extent, but the position of the hands at the end of a finishing technique—provided the technique has accomplished what it set out to do—is merely an aesthetic concern.

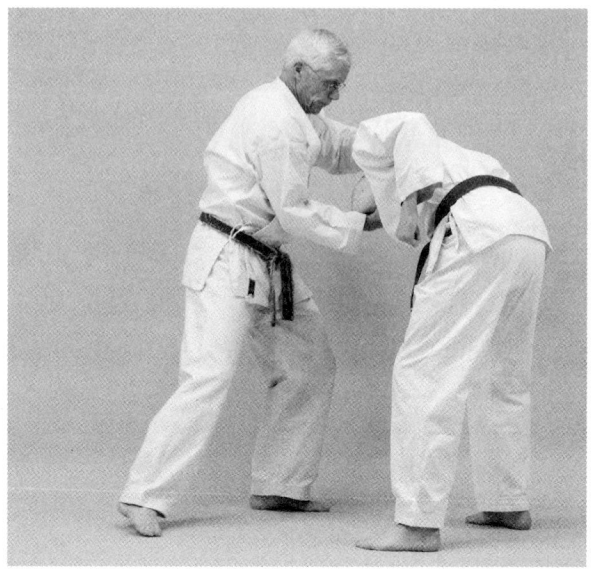

FIGURE 2.71 The simplest way to envision this last technique is to turn to the front, pushing down on the head with the left hand and pulling up on the chin with the right hand.

Most schools, however, will show what looks like an elaborate circling of the arms to finally end up in this last posture with both hands being brought down into the double bent-wrist posture. Or, on occasion, one hand will be brought down into the bent-wrist hand position as the other is brought up. In any case, the circling motion of the hands should begin as the defender is turning to the front, using one's body, not just the arms, to manipulate the opponent. In either case, the left hand is used merely to hold or push down on the opponent's head. The right hand is first pulled back from the spear-hand position, where the right arm was extended under the opponent's throat, in order to grab the attacker's chin. Then, while stepping across and turning to the front, the right hand first pulls up and in on the chin and then rotates around the chin to push out and down (fig. 2.70).

Returning to *Yoi*

See figures 3.61–63.

At the finish of the last sequence, the right foot is brought back to the left foot in what is referred to as musubi dachi, heels together with the feet pointed out at an angle. At the same time, both hands are brought together, the left open palm pressing against the back of the right hand, whether the right hand is open, or closed into a fist as is done in some schools, as the breath is drawn in. Then the hands are rotated, finishing in a downward position in front of the body as the breath is exhaled. If the right fist is used in returning to yoi, then it is generally opened at this point. This position is sometimes held for the count of three breaths in order to calm one's breathing and settle one's mind after the execution of the kata. Then, to finish, the hands are brought alongside the body.

3

KATA: SUPARINPEI

FACING DIRECTIONS WILL BE LABELED with cardinal points north (N), south (S), east (E), and west (W), and ordinal points northwest (NW), southwest (SW), northeast (NE), and southeast (SE). Kata begins facing north (N).

There are some differences in how the various schools of Okinawan Goju-ryu perform Suparinpei kata, but most of these differences are small and insignificant and do not appreciably change how the techniques are applied. This is why, I believe, it is important to understand the applications of kata. Though kata has no doubt undergone some changes in recent years, it is my belief that the differences one might notice in at least the traditional schools of Okinawan karate were based on the manner in which individual teachers sought to accomplish the same thing. That is, at least in my experience, the kata may show slight differences, but the bunkai is the same. The kata I am demonstrating here is the way that I have chosen to do the kata. It is very close to the way I learned the kata almost forty years ago, but I'm sure it's not exactly the same.

One should remember the limitations that still photographs place on kata movement. The temptation, of course, is to see each illustrated position as an end point, capturing a natural break in the action, as it were. This is not the case. Rather, the still photograph, at least in the case of application sequences, provides an unwanted interruption in movements that are often meant to be connected—movement that is meant to be continuous, without gaps. A real understanding of a technique in kata is more often than not revealed only in the movement between each of these still photographs or illustrations.

The still photographs illustrate how we generally teach the movements of the kata. They do not, for the most part, show any of the intermediate movements—how one gets from one position to the next. This, of course, is

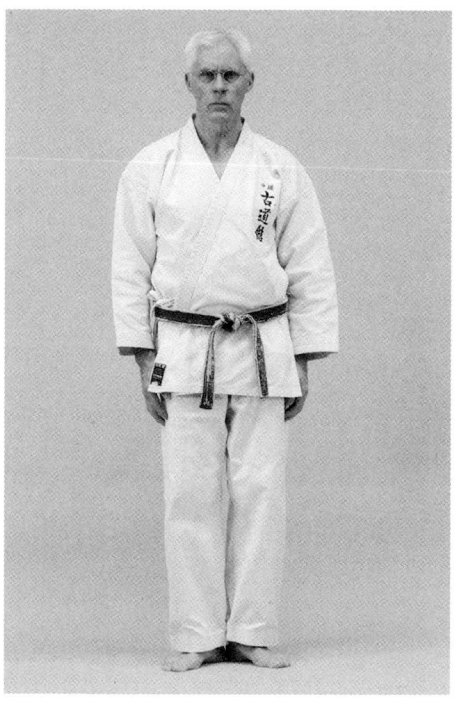

FIGURE 3.1

Feet together in musubi dachi. Attention stance. (N—steps 1 through 25)

one of the unavoidable shortcomings of printed text, regardless of how many still photographs one might include. Additionally, where the kata repeats a series of movements in different directions—as it does in the first half of the kata—I have chosen to illustrate the movements in only one direction, noting the repetition in the caption with the appropriate directional references.

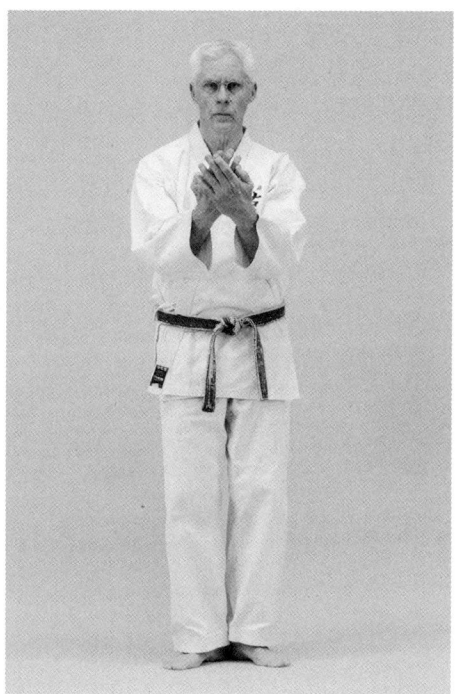

FIGURE 3.2

Feet together in musubi dachi as the hands are brought up, palms facing, in front of the chest, while slowly inhaling through the nose.

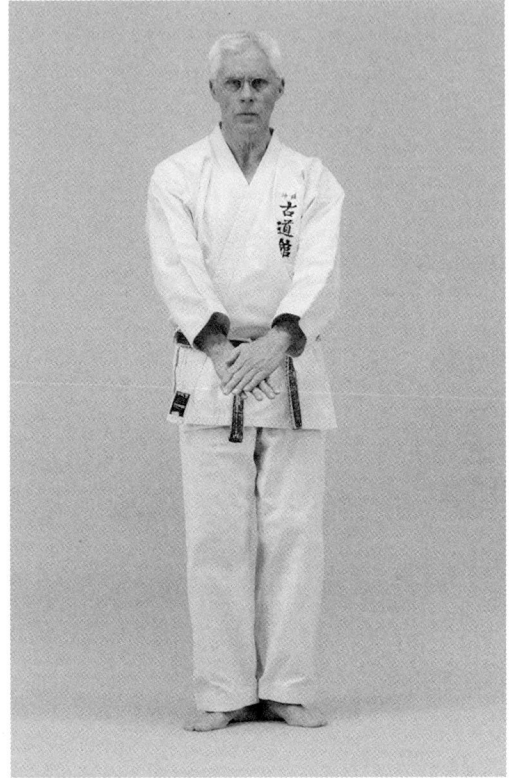

FIGURE 3.3

Feet together in musubi dachi as the hands are rotated and slowly lowered, while slowly exhaling.

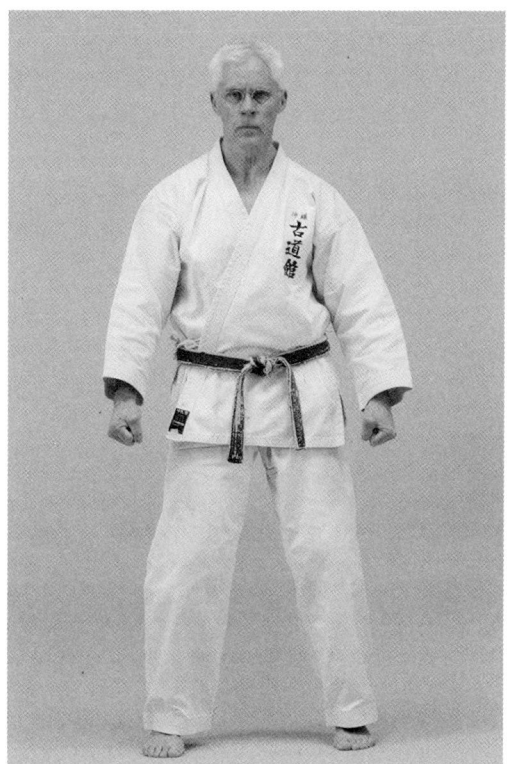

FIGURE 3.4

After the hands are brought together and lowered—the breath drawn in and slowly exhaled, with the attention on the dantian—the hands and feet separate, the hands closed into fists and the feet in heiko dachi, shoulder-width apart.

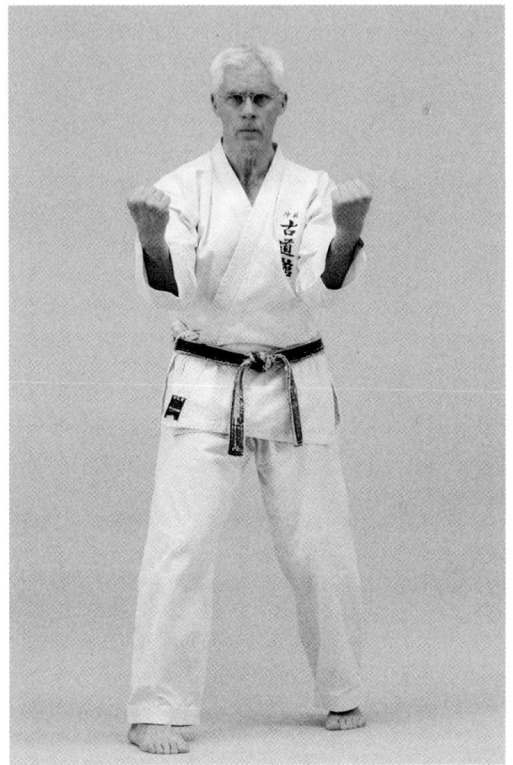

FIGURE 3.5

Stepping into a right-foot-forward sanchin dachi, both arms are brought up into a closed-fist double middle blocking position. This movement and the movements that accompany the next two forward steps are the same as we find in Sanchin kata.

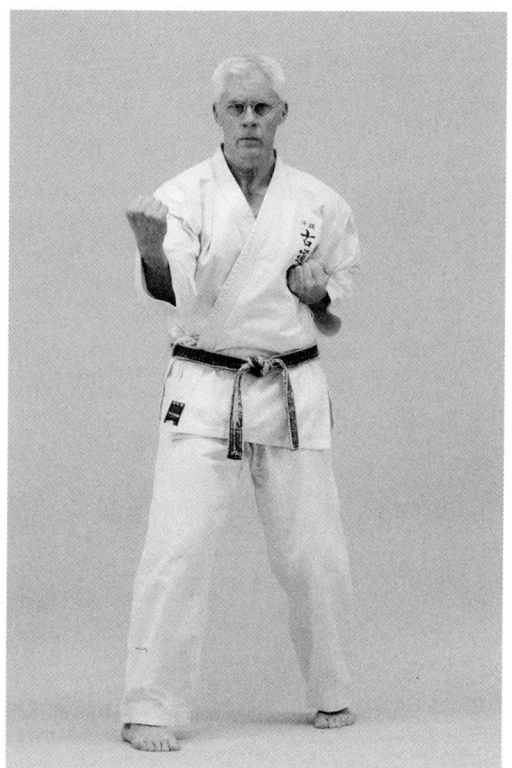

FIGURE 3.6

The left fist is drawn back, alongside the chest—what some refer to as *hiki te* (pulling hand). Each of these three beginning "punches" is preceded by this drawing-in motion.

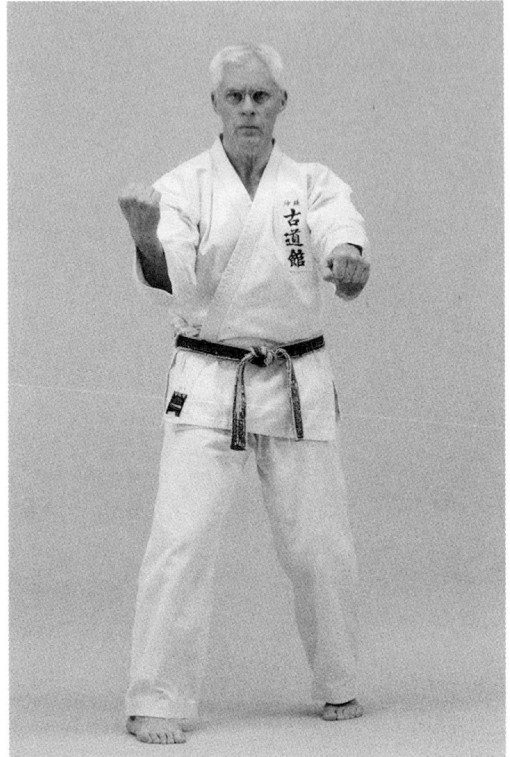

FIGURE 3.7

After the fist is drawn back, it is slowly extended. The "punches" are executed straight out, in front of the shoulder but at middle-level height. The
breath is drawn in as the fist is drawn back and slowly exhaled as the fist
is thrust out.

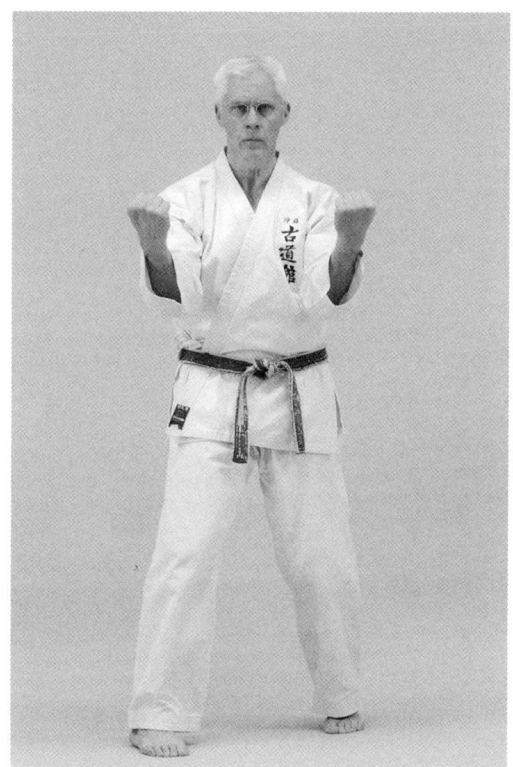

FIGURE 3.8

The fist is then drawn back, the elbow dropping, into the middle blocking, or kamae, position. This is executed with a short inhale and exhale of breath.

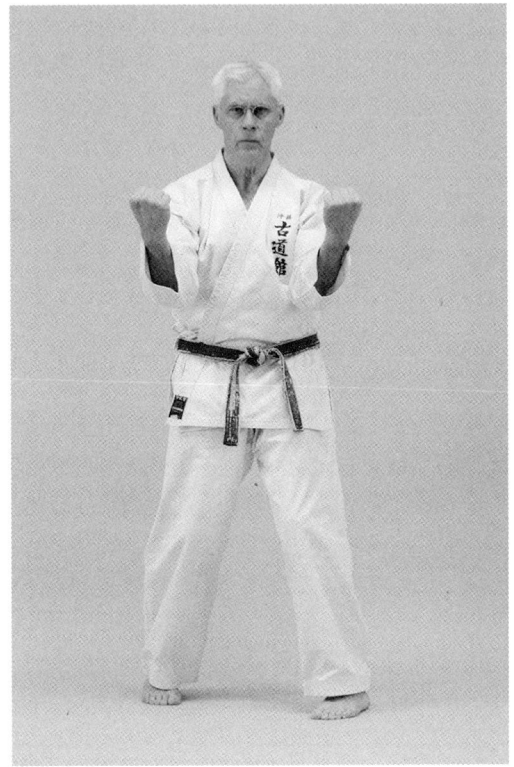

FIGURE 3.9

Step into a left-foot-forward sanchin dachi. Goju-ryu kata generally employs a crescent step in moving forward or back in sanchin dachi.

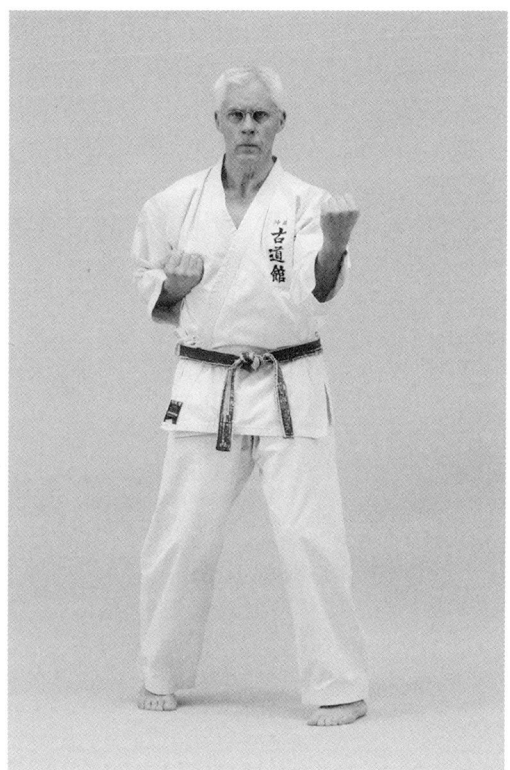

FIGURE 3.10

The right fist is drawn back, alongside the chest. This is the same movement as we see in figure 3.6, above, executed on the left side. Again, the breath is coordinated with the movement of the arms, along with a slight sinking feeling and rotation of the waist.

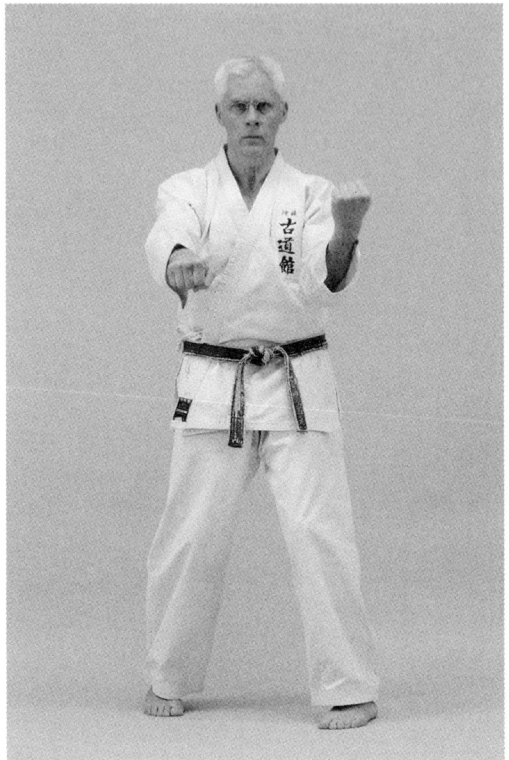

FIGURE 3.11

The right fist is slowly extended as the breath is exhaled. One should have the feeling that the whole body is connected to this movement, that the movement of the arm originates in the legs and waist.

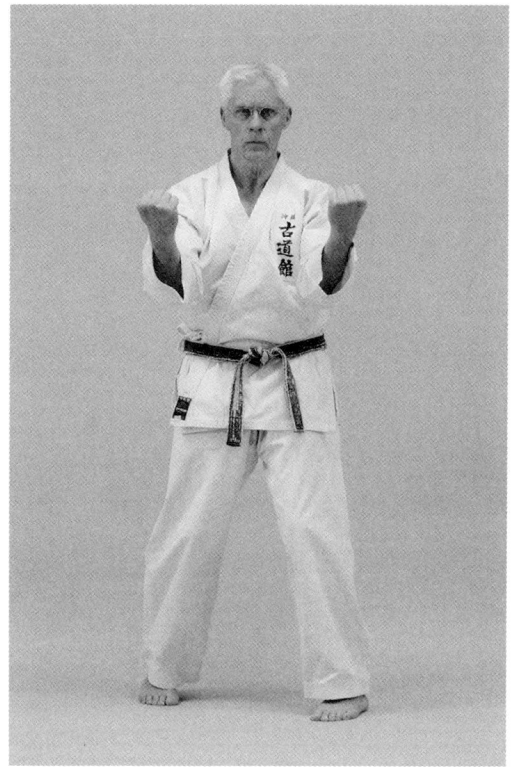

FIGURE 3.12

The fist is drawn back, the elbow dropping, into the middle blocking, or kamae, position. Again, this is executed with a short inhale and exhale of breath.

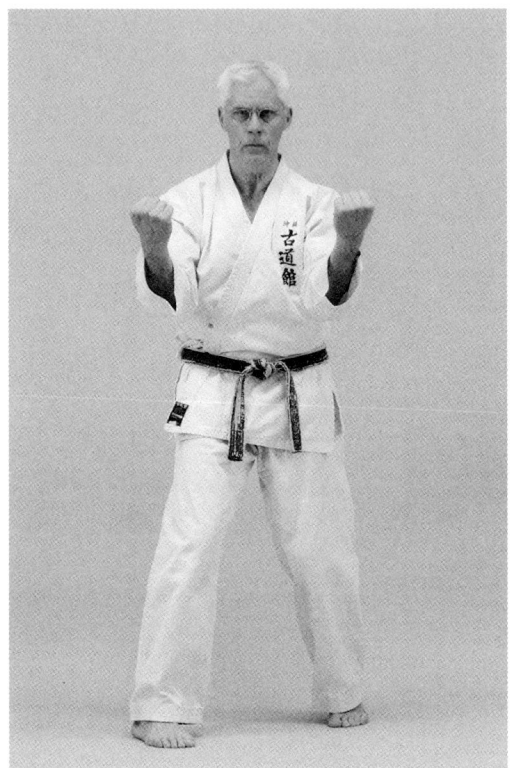

FIGURE 3.13

Step into a right-foot-forward sanchin dachi.

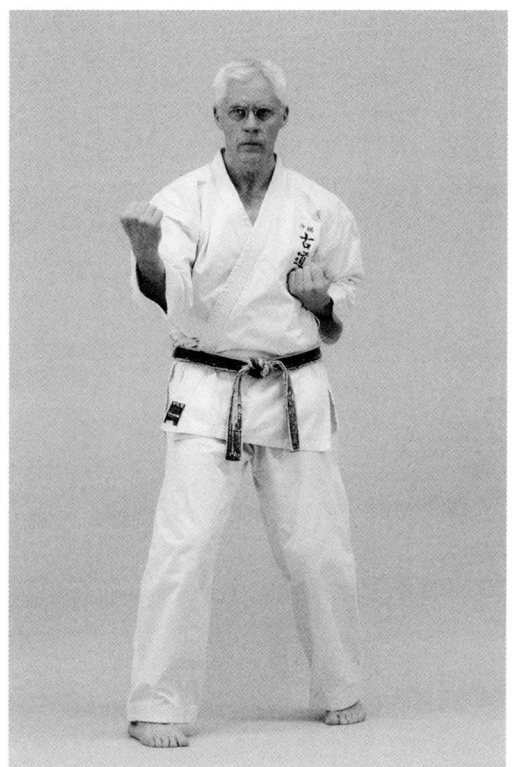

FIGURE 3.14

The left fist is drawn back, alongside the chest, repeating the movements we see in figure 3.6, above.

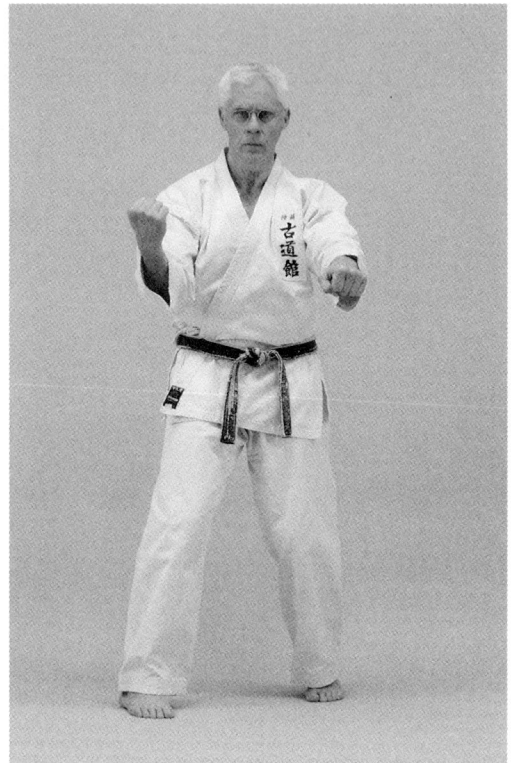

FIGURE 3.15

The left fist is slowly extended as the breath is exhaled.

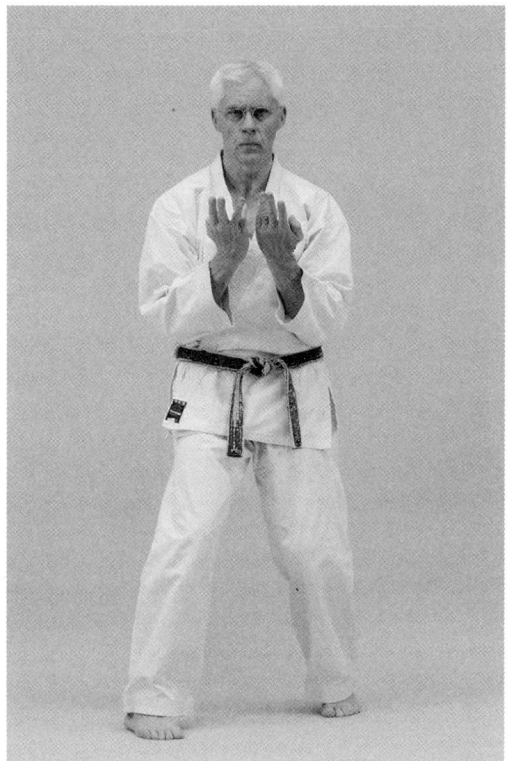

FIGURE 3.16

Sinking slightly with both knees bent, the hands open and are drawn in toward the center of the chest.

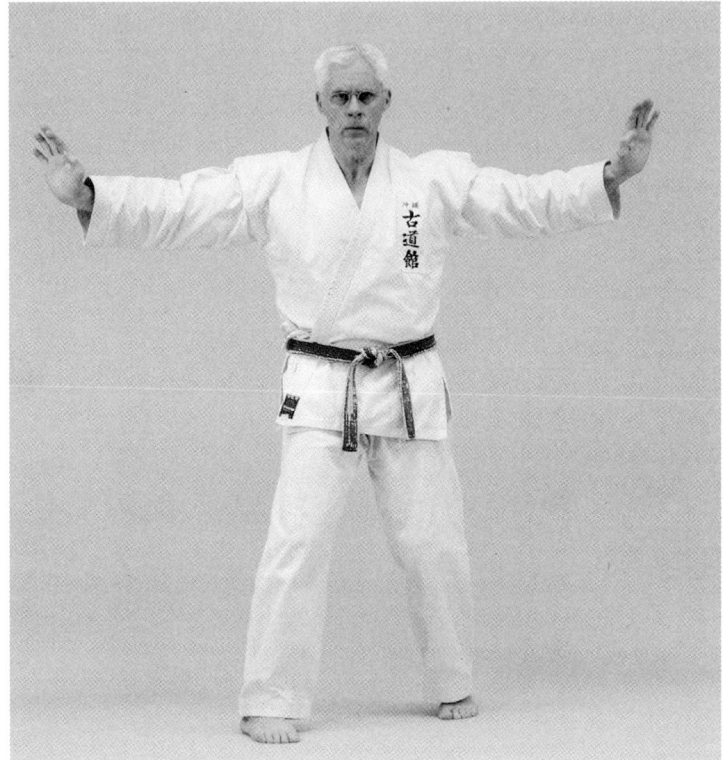

FIGURE 3.17

Both hands are then thrust out to the side, palms out, shoulder height.

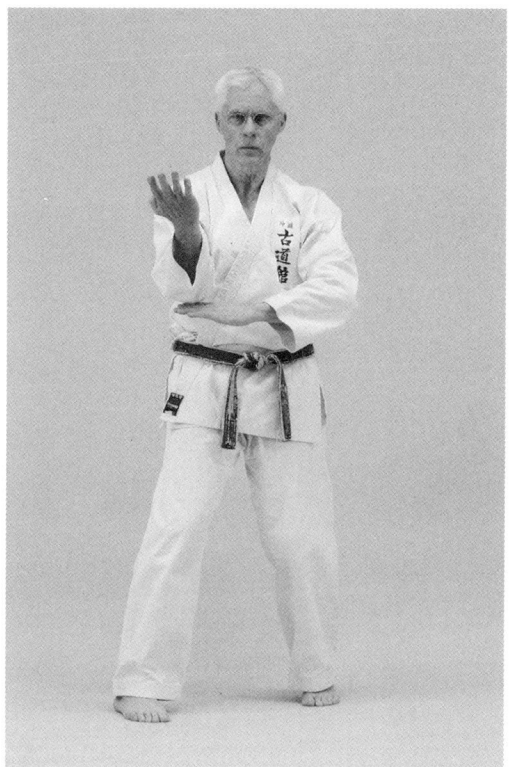

FIGURE 3.18

The right forearm is brought in, with the arm bent and the elbow down, as the left hand is brought across the body at waist level, just under the right elbow or forearm. Both hands remain open, with the right hand palm-up and the left hand palm-down. This is not a fixed position, but a movement that precedes each of the mawashi uke, though the hands will be reversed for the left mawashi uke, and usually performed in conjunction with the forward step—that is, the hands and feet move together. This series, movements 18 through 25, is repeated three more times: first to the south, then to the east, and then to the west.

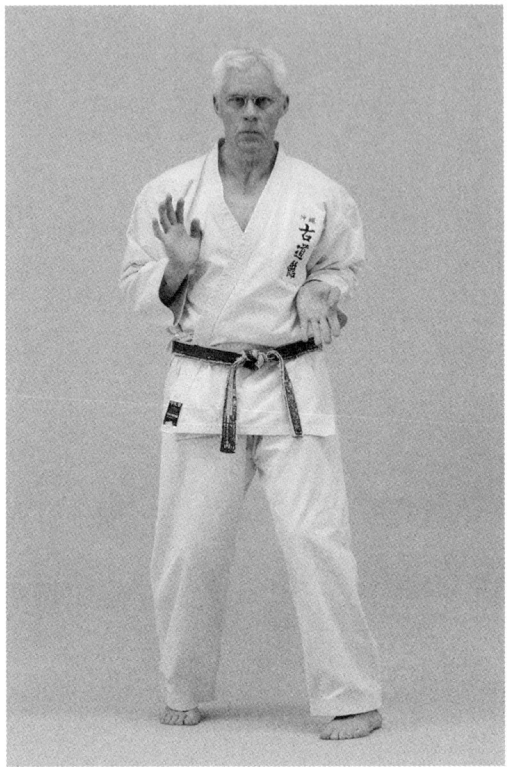

FIGURE 3.19

Step forward into a left-foot-forward sanchin dachi and perform a right mawashi uke. In the right mawashi uke, the right arm pushes in toward the center as the left hand is brought across the body and under the right arm (fig. 3.18). Both arms then move in a circular fashion, counterclockwise. Traditionally, the hands are drawn in, alongside the chest, with the right hand palm forward, pointing up, and the left hand palm forward, pointing down. This position is illustrated here, though in reality the pulling-in and pushing-out motion of the mawashi uke is probably exaggerated and should not be seen as a separate technique.

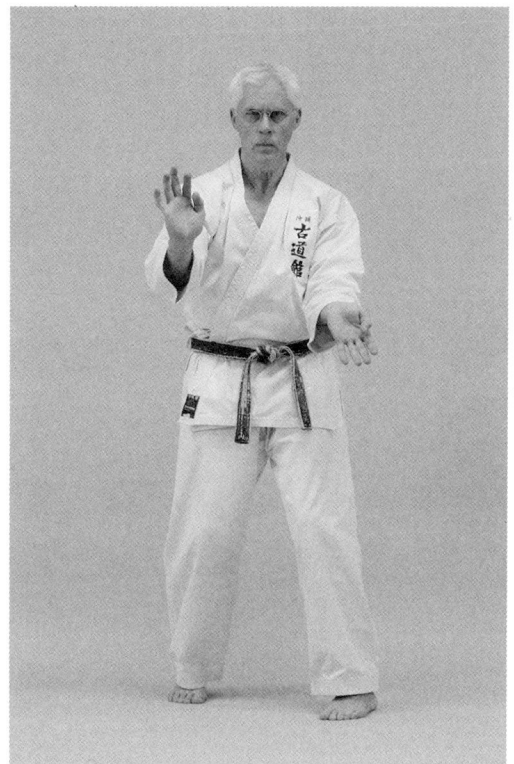

FIGURE 3.20

As one sinks into the forward step, the hands push out.

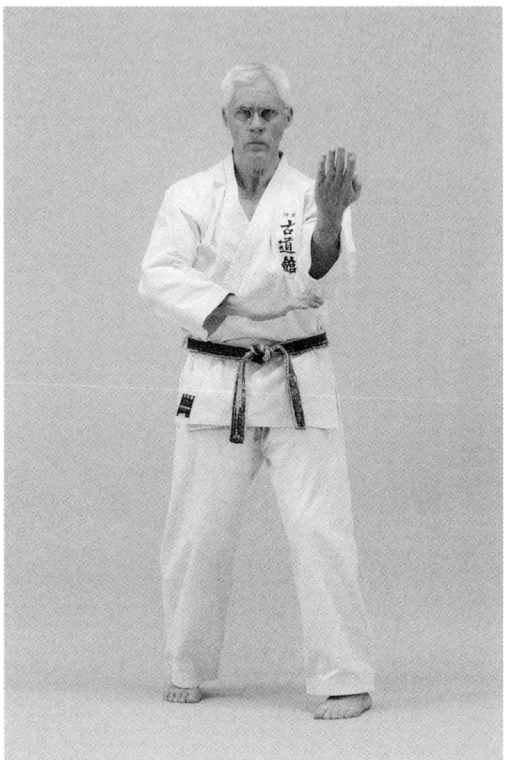

FIGURE 3.21

Following the right mawashi uke, the left forearm is brought up, with the arm bent and the elbow down, as the right hand is brought across the body at waist level, just under the left elbow or forearm. Both hands remain open, with the right hand palm-down and the left hand palm-up. Again, this is not a fixed position, and should accompany the step into a right-foot-forward sanchin dachi.

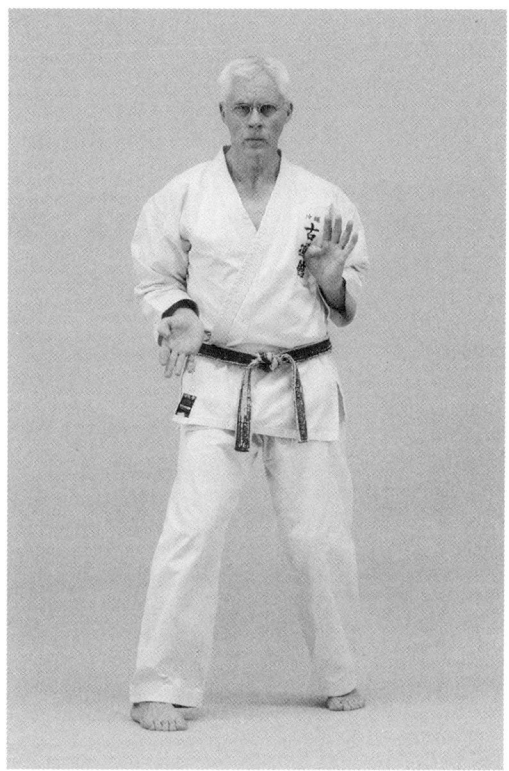

FIGURE 3.22

Stepping forward into a right-foot-forward sanchin dachi, perform a left mawashi uke, both arms moving in a circular fashion, clockwise, ending with the palms forward, the left hand pointing up and the right hand pointing down. Just as in the right mawashi uke, the movements are coordinated, and the hands seem to pull in as the circular motion of the arms is completed.

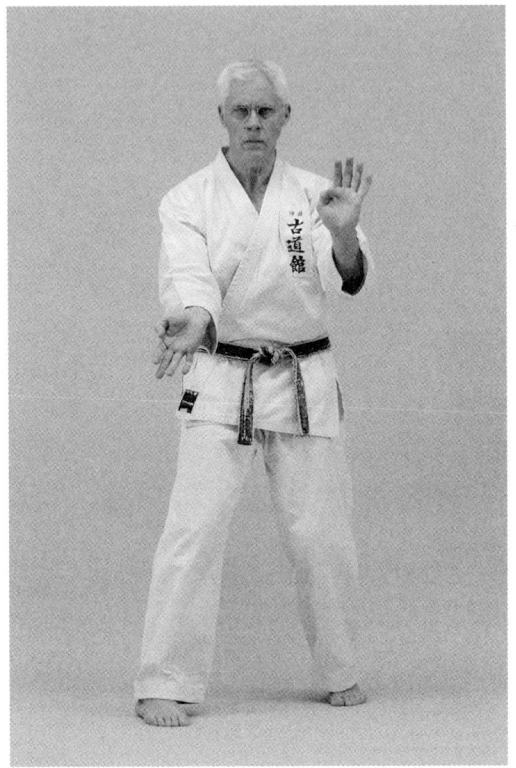

FIGURE 3.23

As one sinks into the forward step, the hands push out.

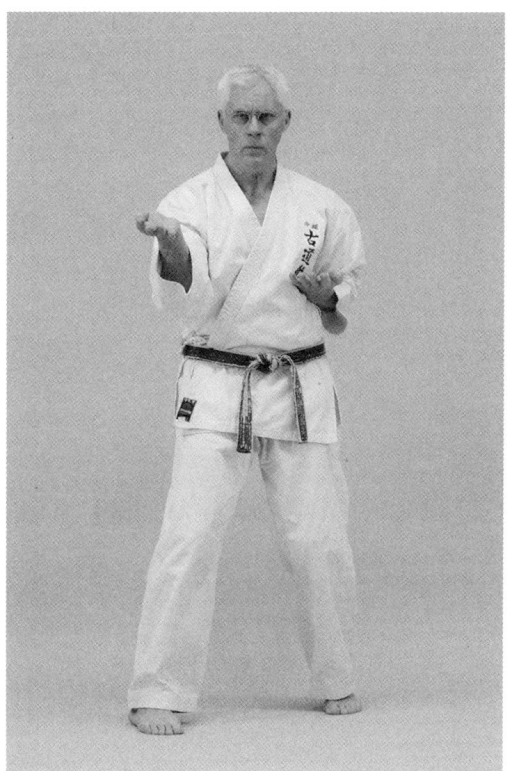

FIGURE 3.24

The right hand is brought up, making sure to keep the elbow down, as the left hand is brought back to the side of the chest. Raising the hand while keeping the elbow down is an important concept here. In reality, there would be no pause between this movement and the movements depicted in figure 3.25.

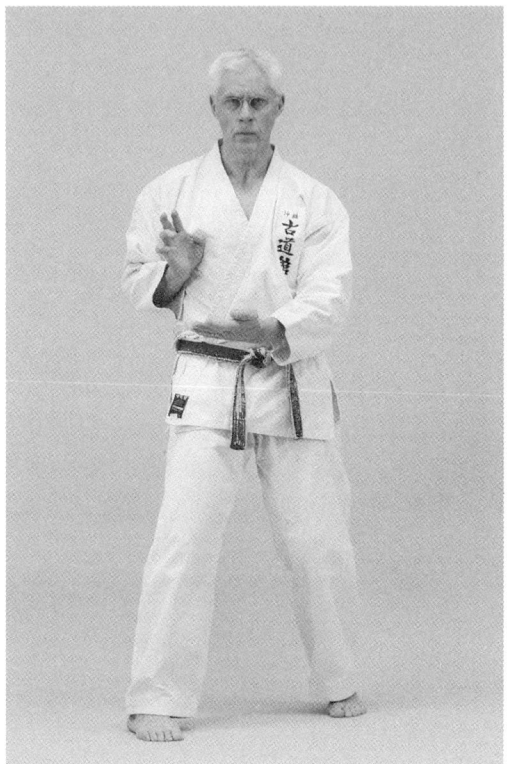

FIGURE 3.25

The right hand is first rotated, palm forward, and then pulled in, as the left open hand is thrust out. In application, this technique is connected to the first (right) mawashi uke technique. The right hand is on the opponent's head and the left hand is used to attack the throat and control the chin (see fig. 2.15 for application). This series of techniques, steps 18 through 25, is repeated three more times: First, with a 180-degree counterclockwise turn to the south; then, a 90-degree counterclockwise turn to the east; and finally, a 180-degree counterclockwise turn to the west. The last of the double mawashi uke and nukite/shuto series of techniques is performed facing west.

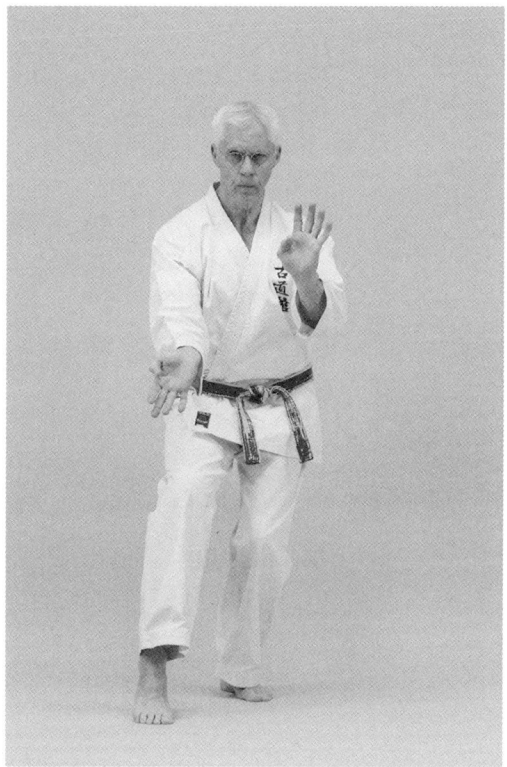

FIGURE 3.26

Shifting back into a right-foot-forward Cat Stance, after the last of the double mawashi uke and nukite/shuto combinations, facing west, the hands circle (clockwise) in a mawashi-like manner, similar to the technique we see at the end of Saifa kata or in the middle of Kururunfa kata. In the final position, the left hand is pointed up, palm forward, and the right hand is pointed down, palm forward. (W)

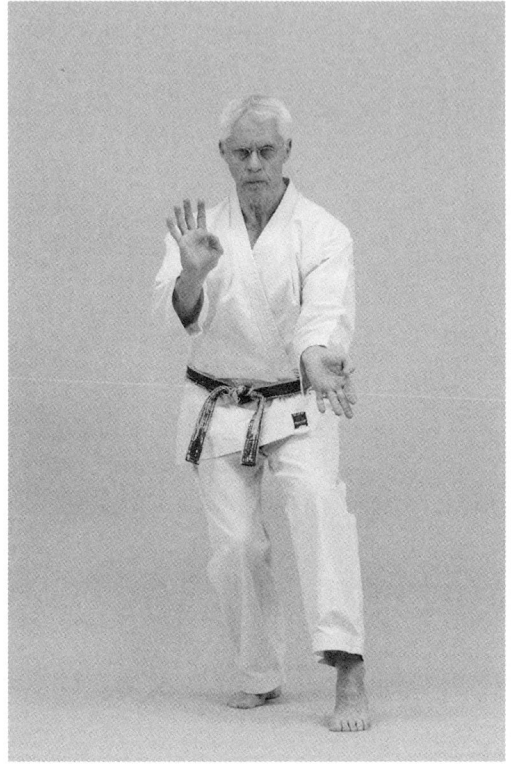

FIGURE 3.27

This technique repeats, on the opposite side (counterclockwise), with a 180-degree turn to the left (east) into a left-foot-forward Cat Stance. (E)

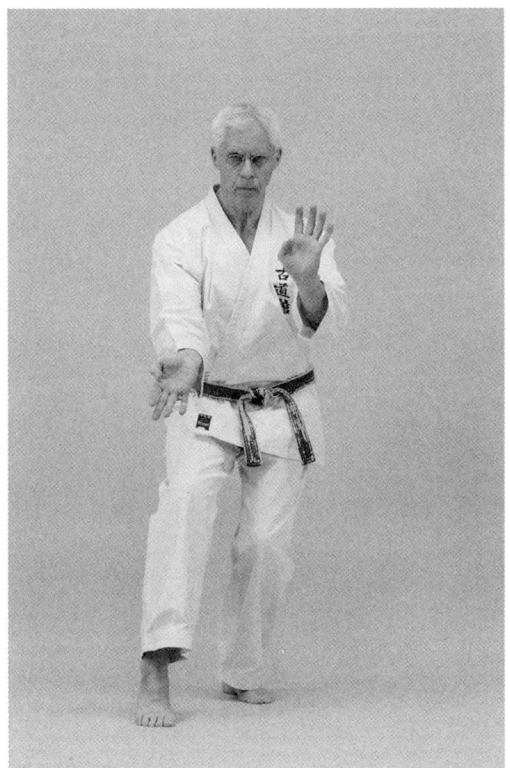

FIGURE 3.28

The technique repeats, on the first illustrated side (repeating step 26 above), with a 90-degree turn to the right (south) into a right-foot-forward Cat Stance. (S)

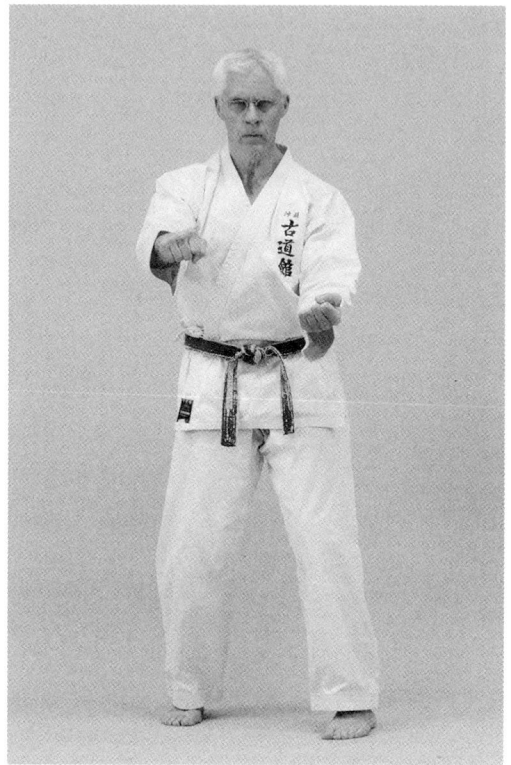

FIGURE 3.29

Turning counterclockwise 180 degrees to the original front (N) into a left-foot-forward sanchin dachi, both hands close and are first drawn in—the pulling-in coordinated with the turn—and then thrust out in what is conventionally referred to as a double punch. It is important to keep in mind here, and each time this technique is repeated, that the hands are first open and then closed (see fig. 2.30 for application). (N—steps 29 through 31)

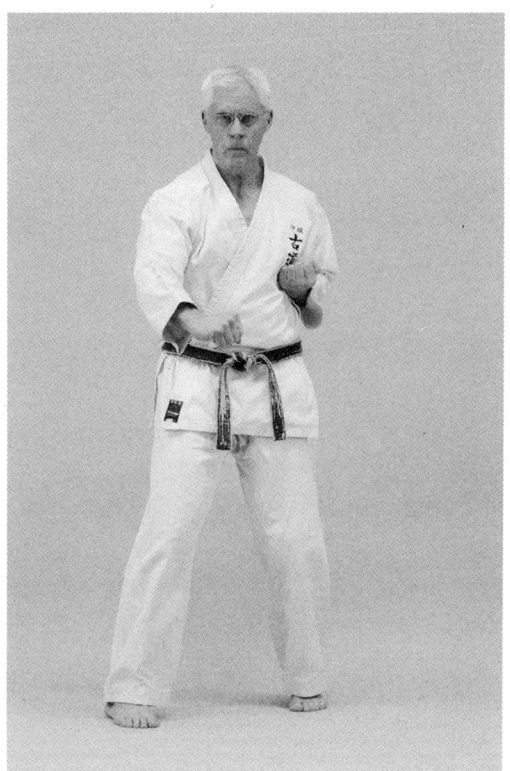

FIGURE 3.30

Stepping forward into a right sanchin dachi, the right arm pushes (or pulls) down. The movement of the right arm, conventionally referred to as a blocking or parrying technique, generally precedes the left "punch."

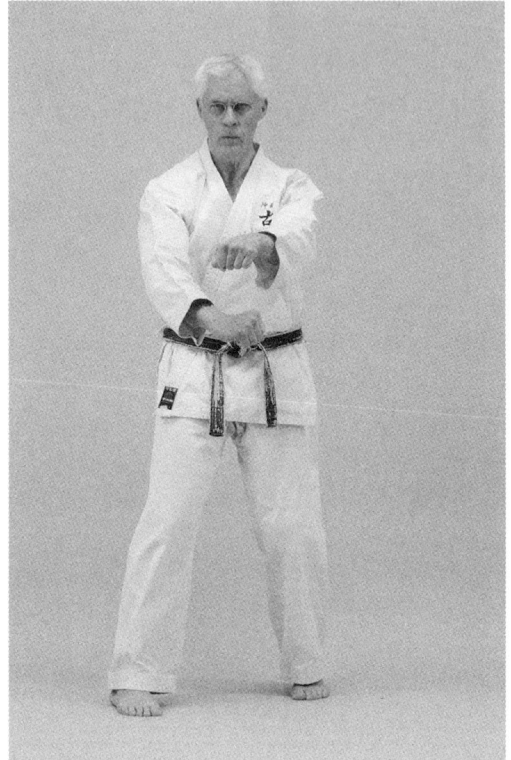

FIGURE 3.31

The left fist is then thrust out over the right arm. The speed of the "punch" often varies in the performance of kata, as well as the timing between the execution of the blocking or parrying technique and the "punch." This series of techniques, steps 29 through 31, is repeated three more times: First, with a 180-degree counterclockwise turn to the south; then, a 90-degree counterclockwise turn to the east; and finally, a 180-degree counterclockwise turn to the west.

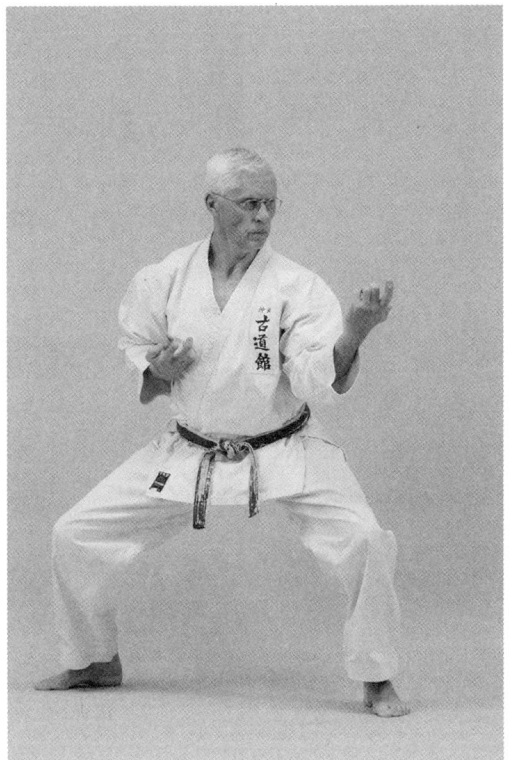

FIGURE 3.32

After the last of the double punch, parry, and left middle-level punch combinations, facing west, the right foot steps out to the northwest (NW),
dropping into shiko dachi, as the left arm is rotated, elbow down and
palm up, with the fingers slightly curled. The right hand is open or partially closed, palm up, in front of the chest. The attention is directed to the
southeast corner. The feet are positioned along the southeast–northwest
axis, slightly offset, with the left foot to the southeast and the right foot to
the northwest (see fig. 2.33 for application). (View of kata here is from the
southwest.) (SE—steps 32 through 34)

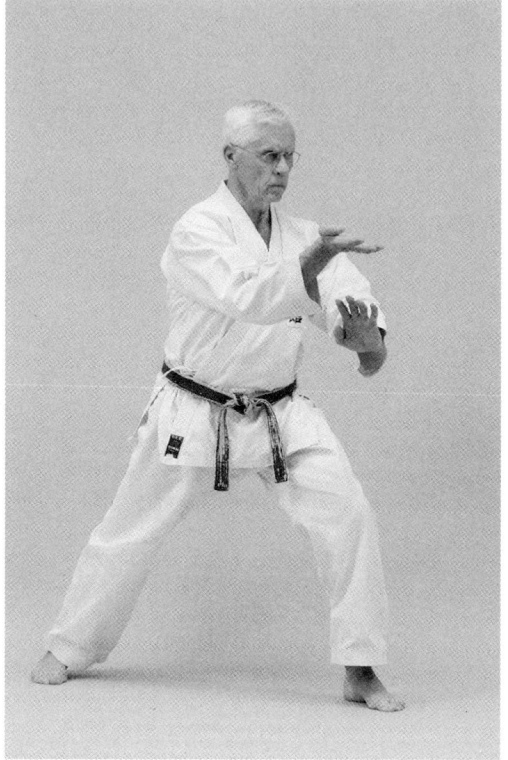

FIGURE 3.33

Momentarily shifting to a left-foot-forward Front Stance, the left hand rotates as the right hand is thrust out in the direction of the southeast corner. This is transitional and should not be seen as a stopping point.

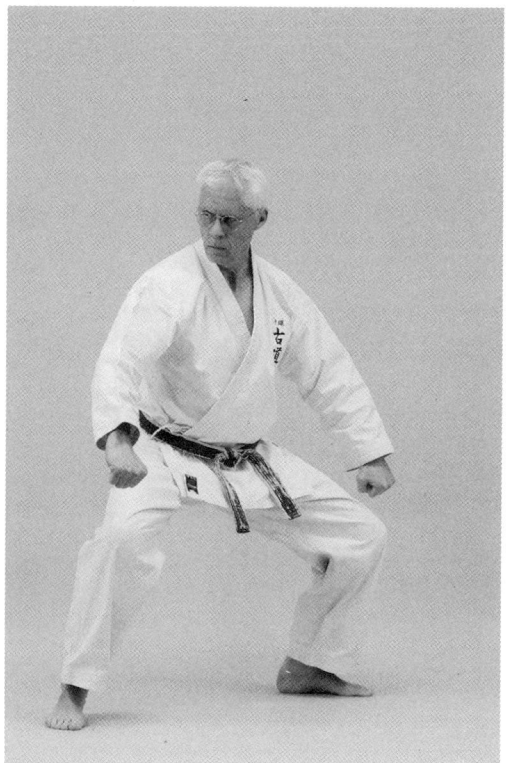

FIGURE 3.34

Stepping with the right foot to the southeast corner into shiko dachi, both arms are brought down, hands closed, into what is conventionally referred to as a double low block. (View of kata here is from the northeast.) This series of techniques, steps 32 through 34, is repeated three more times: First, with a 180-degree counterclockwise turn to face the northwest; then, bringing the right foot back, a 90-degree counterclockwise turn to face the southwest; and finally, a 180-degree counterclockwise turn to face the northeast.

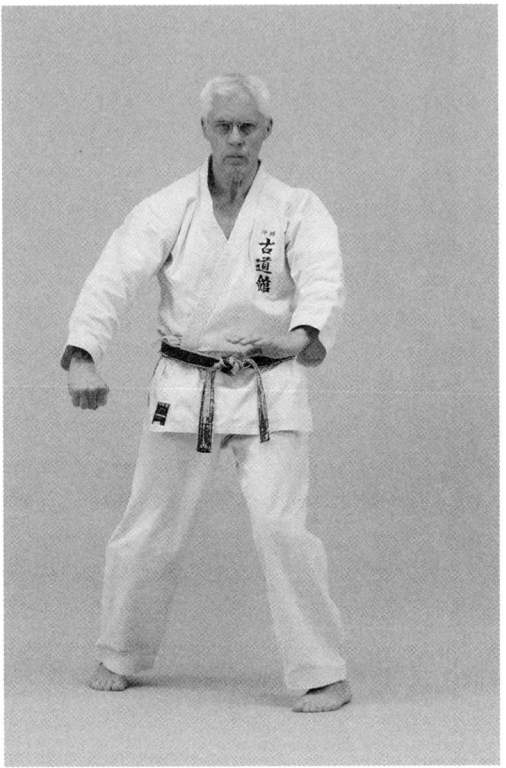

FIGURE 3.35

The second half of the kata—and the first complete sequence—begins after the last of the four shiko dachi angle techniques. Step up toward the original front (N) with first the left foot, as the left arm is brought around in a clockwise semicircular motion, the open hand ending in the down position (see fig. 2.35 for application). (N—steps 35 through 42)

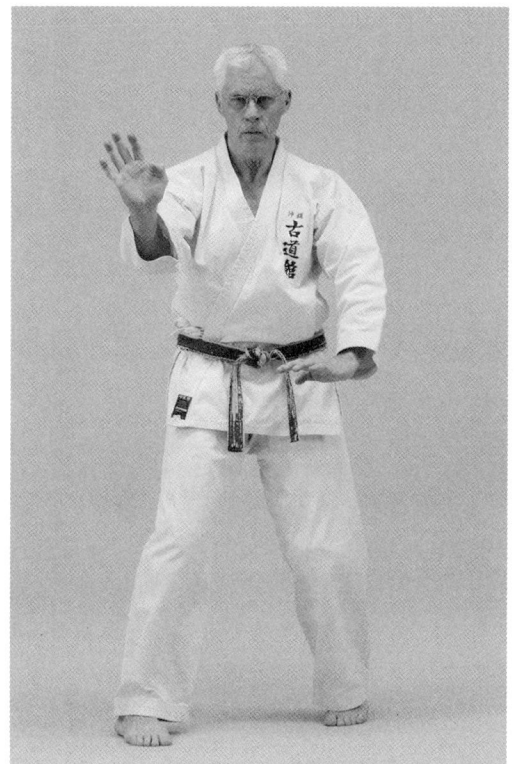

FIGURE 3.36

Then step forward with the right foot, as the right arm is brought up in a clockwise semicircular motion, ending in a right-foot-forward sanchin dachi (see fig. 2.36 for application).

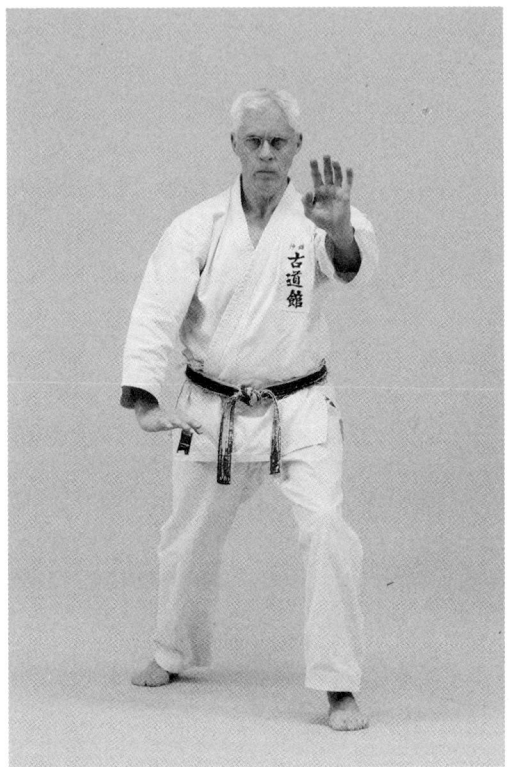

FIGURE 3.37

Step forward into a left-foot-forward Front Stance as the left arm is brought up, left palm forward, and the right arm is brought down, right palm down, into a posture reminiscent of Shisochin kata. Some schools will execute this step in a left-foot-forward Basic Stance with the arms blocking in a manner reminiscent of the Gekisai kata open-hand blocks.

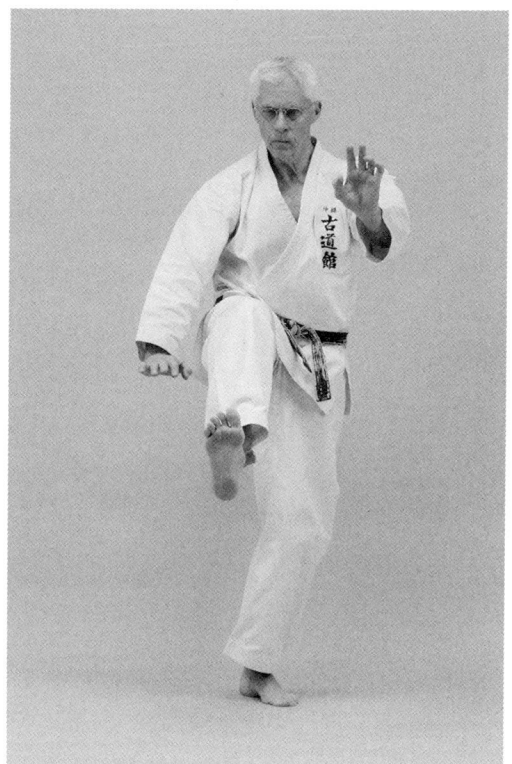

FIGURE 3.38

Kick mae geri with the right foot. In all likelihood, this kick should be directed at the opponent's legs, or at the very least, below the waist (see fig. 2.45 for application).

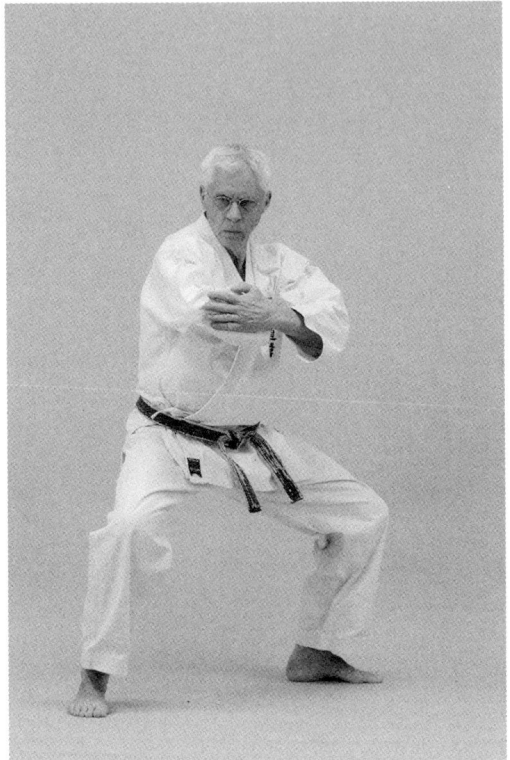

FIGURE 3.39

As the foot is brought down into a right-foot-forward shiko dachi, the right elbow is brought into the left palm, the left hand pulling in as the right elbow is thrust out.

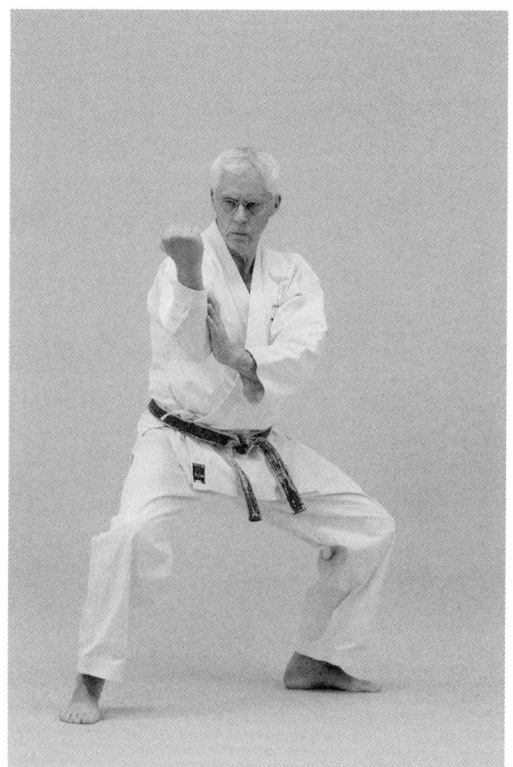

FIGURE 3.40

The right arm "unfolds," with the left hand along the right forearm.

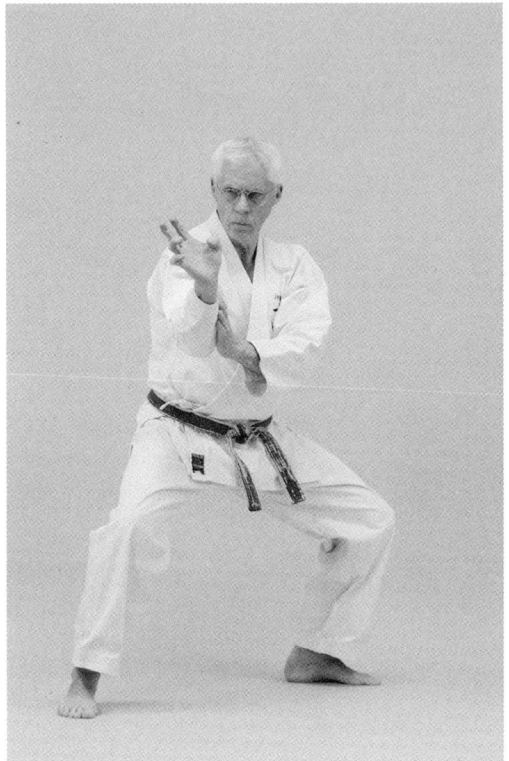

FIGURE 3.41

The right hand opens as it is turned forward. The opening of the right hand signifies the grabbing of the opponent's hair or, in olden days, the topknot, and should be executed in conjunction with the following movement (see fig. 2.50 for application).

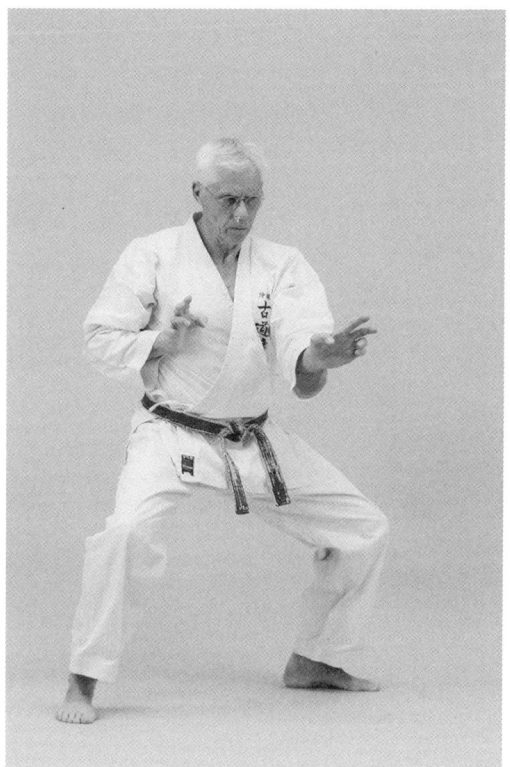

FIGURE 3.42

The right hand is then pulled back as the left open hand is thrust out. What may seem uncharacteristic of Okinawan karate in this technique is that the thumb of the left hand wraps around the right forearm as it pushes out. This is because the left hand is used to push out against the opponent's chin.

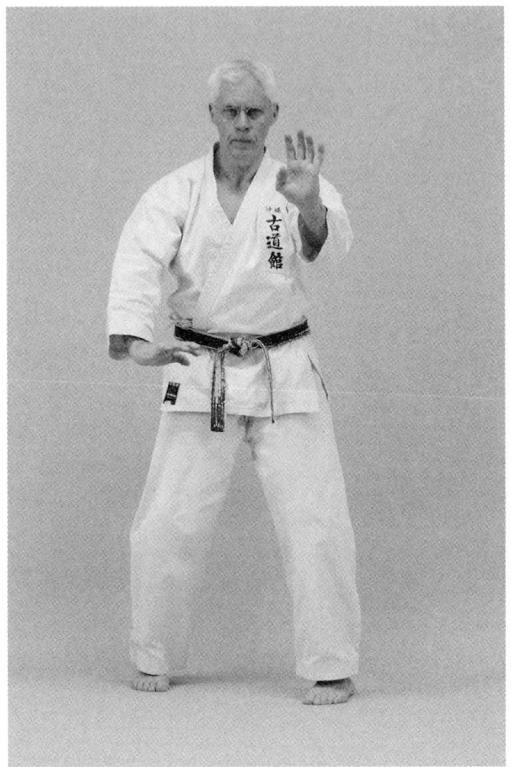

FIGURE 3.43

The right foot steps across into a left-foot-forward sanchin dachi facing south. At the same time, the right arm moves in a semicircular counter-clockwise motion from outside to inside, ending in the down position. The left arm moves up in a semicircular counterclockwise motion from inside to outside, ending in the upper position. (S—steps 43 through 48)

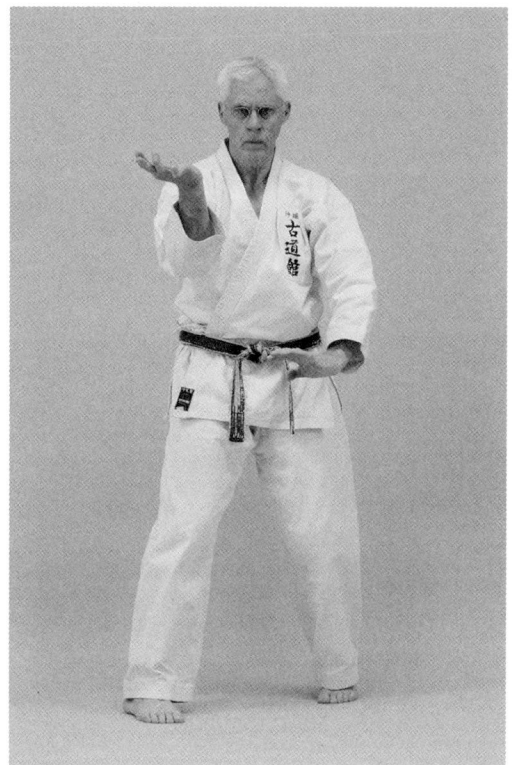

FIGURE 3.44

Stepping forward into a right sanchin dachi, the left hand is brought down and the right hand is brought up.

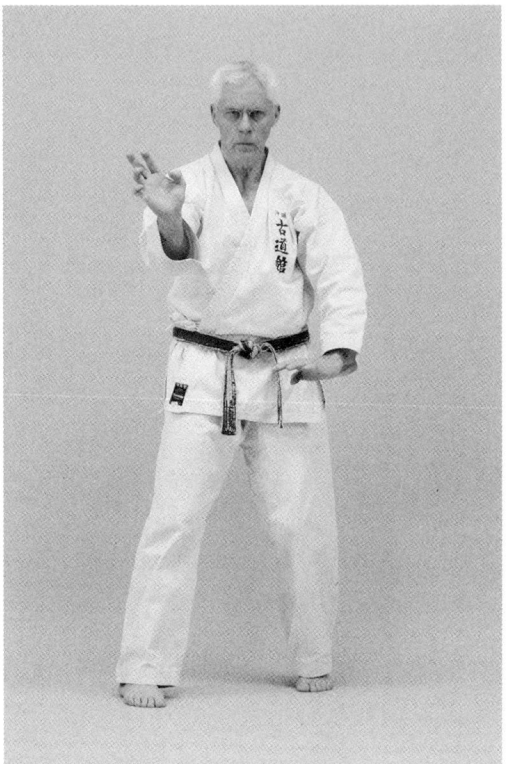

FIGURE 3.45

The right hand is rotated, palm forward. In application, the palms rotate as they change—that is, along with the forward step—as the hand is brought up, the palm rotates up, and as the hand is brought down, the palm rotates down. In the performance of kata, the movements illustrated in steps 44 and 45, and again in steps 46 and 47, are generally separated. However, the stops we usually see in the performance of these steps are artificial and would not occur in the application of the techniques.

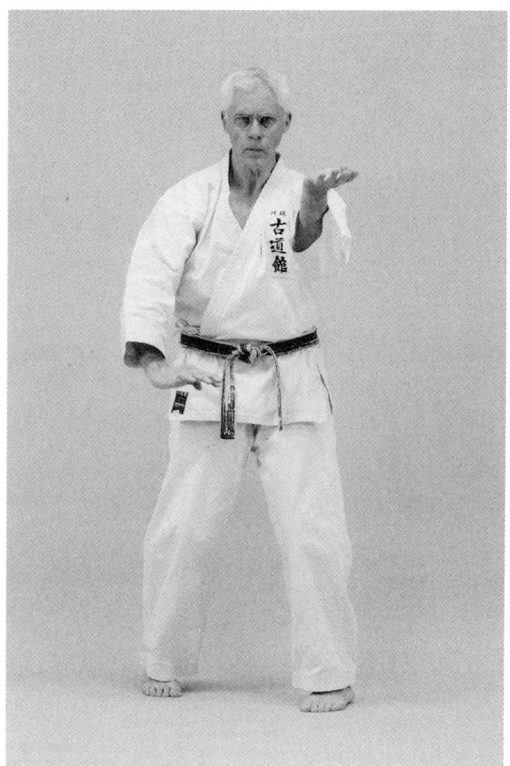

FIGURE 3.46

Stepping forward into a left sanchin dachi, the right hand is brought down and the left hand is brought up.

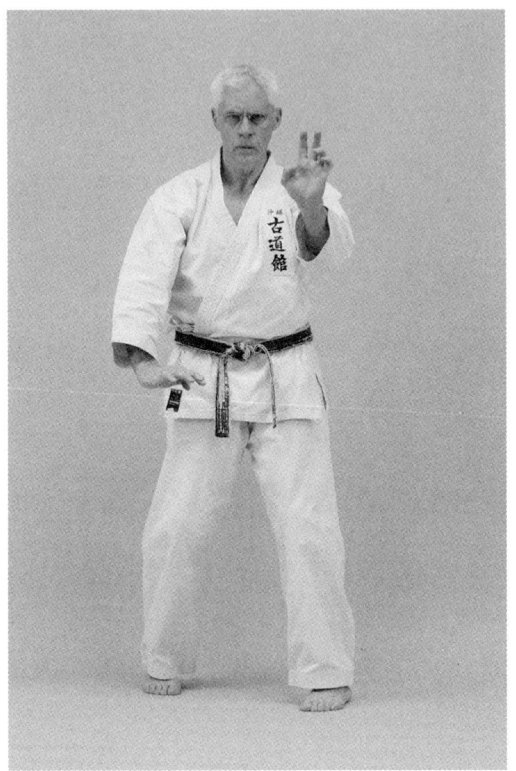

FIGURE 3.47

The left hand is rotated, palm forward.

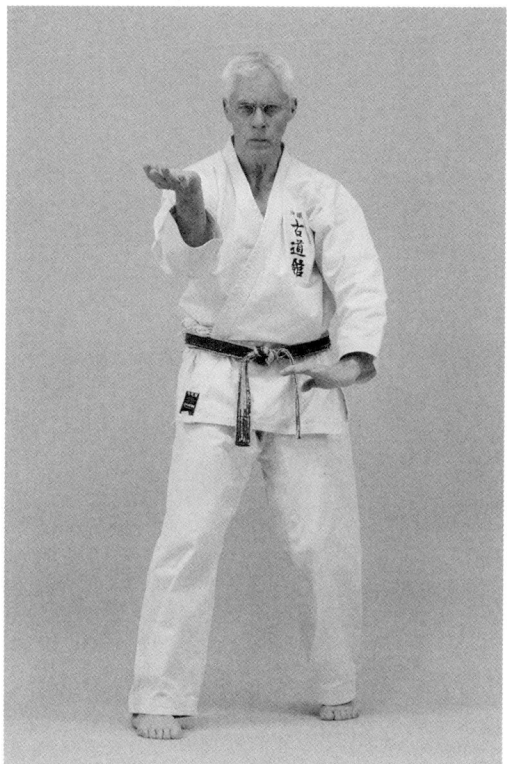

FIGURE 3.48

Stepping forward into a right sanchin dachi, the left hand is brought down and the right hand is brought up.

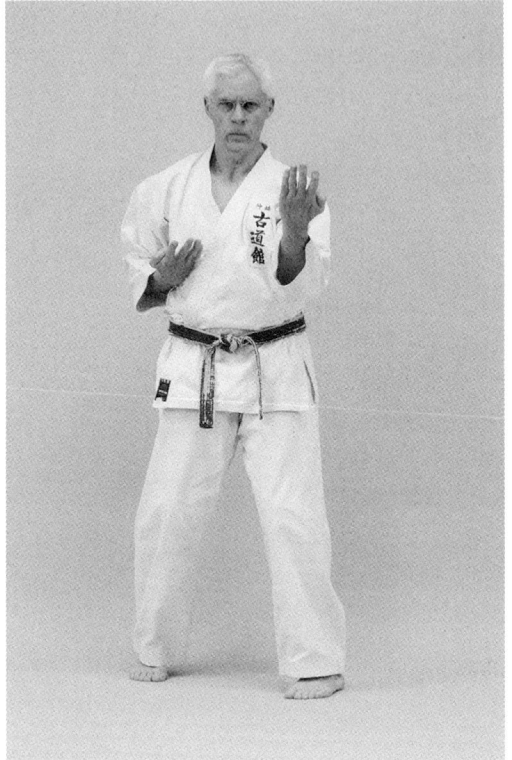

FIGURE 3.49

Stepping across with the right foot, pivot into a left-foot-forward sanchin dachi facing the original front (N). At the same time, the right arm sweeps across the body, ending palm-up along the ribs, and the left arm is brought around in what appears to be a palm-up middle-level block, similar to what we see at the beginning of the third sequence of Kururunfa kata. Again, the pause that we see in the kata performance of this technique would not occur in the application of the technique, since it is part of the sequence of movements depicted in steps 43 through 51 (N).

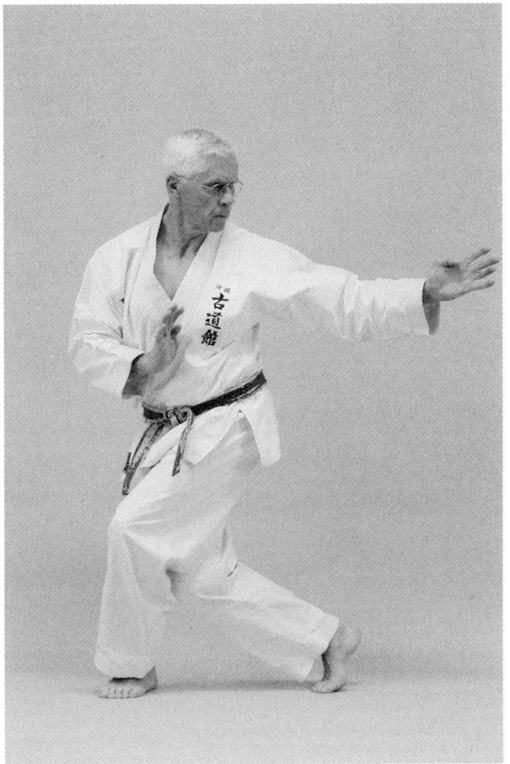

FIGURE 3.50

Pivoting to the left, facing more or less south, the left arm is straightened out, rotating the hand, as the right hand is brought to the center of the chest. (S—steps 50 and 51)

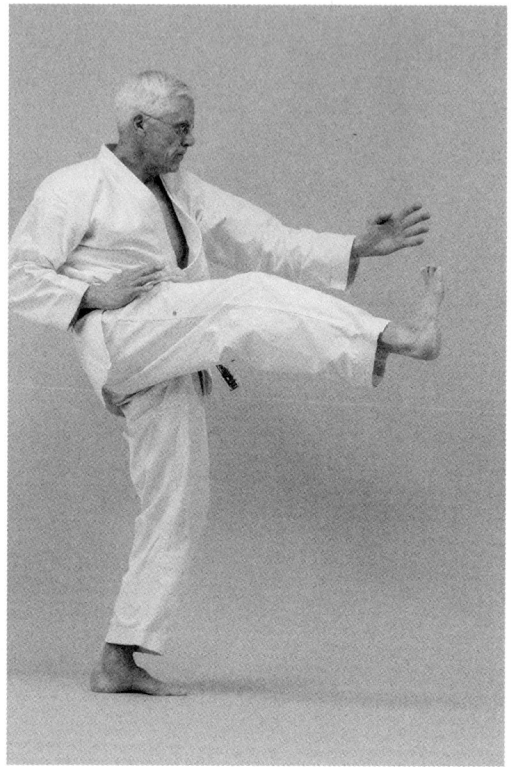

FIGURE 3.51

The right foot or knee is brought around in a large arcing motion to kick at the level of the left hand.

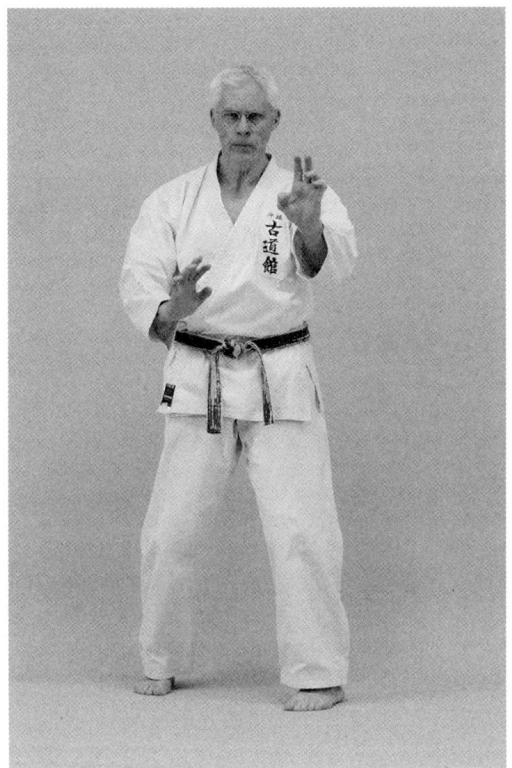

FIGURE 3.52

At the completion of the kick, the right foot is planted, pivoting into a left-foot-forward sanchin dachi, facing the original front, with both hands up. (N—steps 52 through 56)

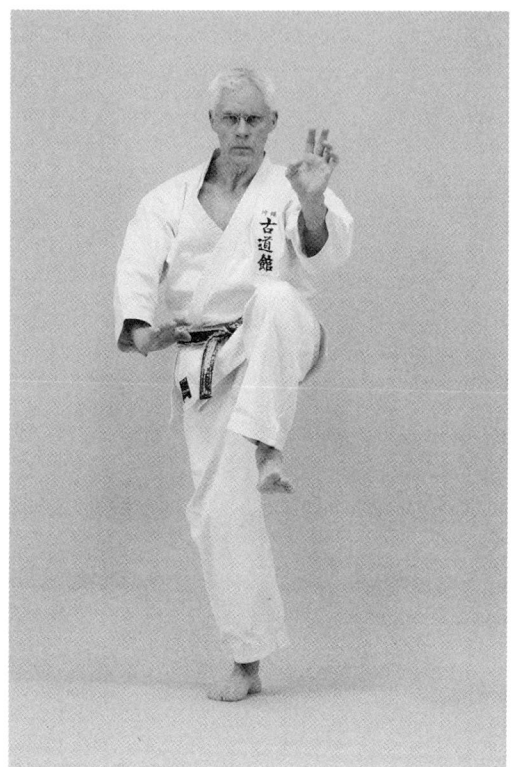

FIGURE 3.53

Pushing off with the right foot, the left knee is raised.

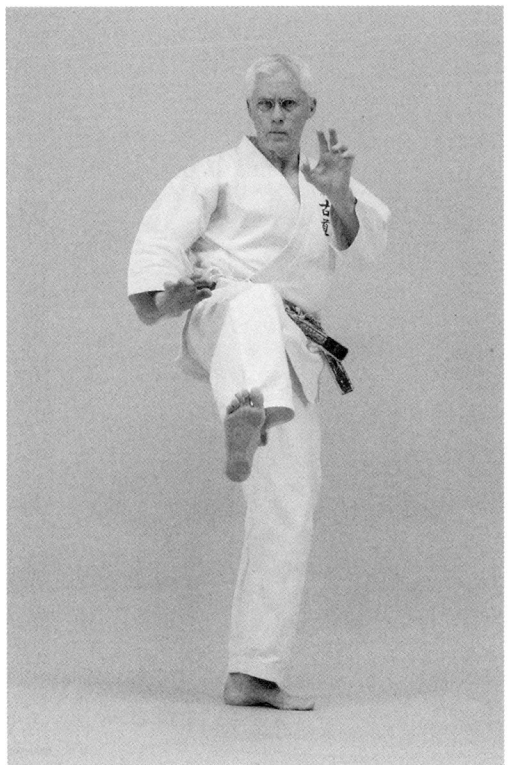

FIGURE 3.54

This raised knee is immediately followed by a right kick while in the air, though this is difficult to capture in a still photograph.

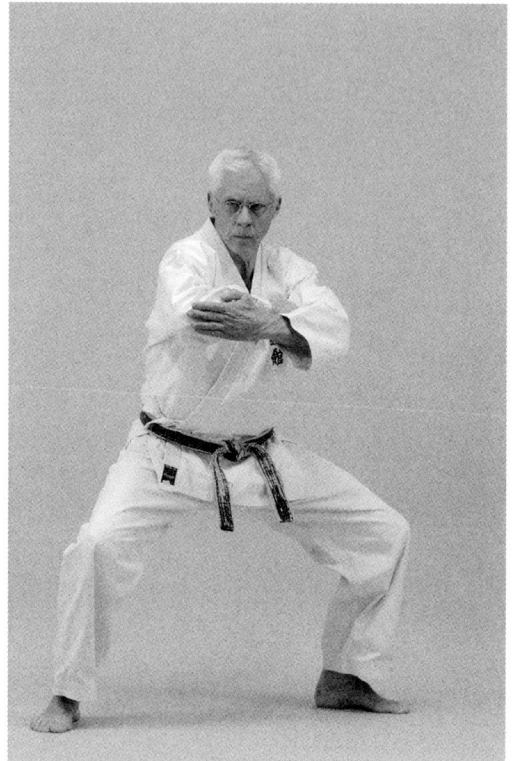

FIGURE 3.55

After the completion of the kick, the right foot is brought down into a right-foot-forward shiko dachi. At the same time, the right elbow is brought into the left palm (see fig. 2.63 for application). This position looks the same as position 39 of the first complete sequence.

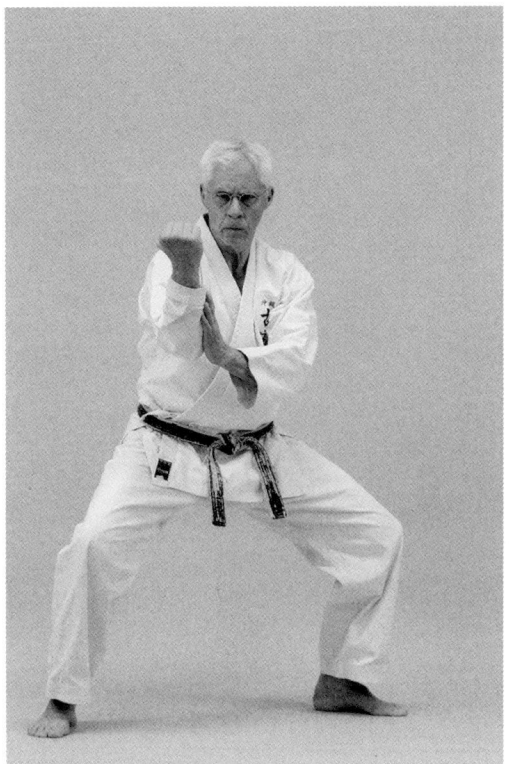

FIGURE 3.56

The right arm "unfolds," with the left hand positioned along the right forearm. This position looks the same as step 40 above.

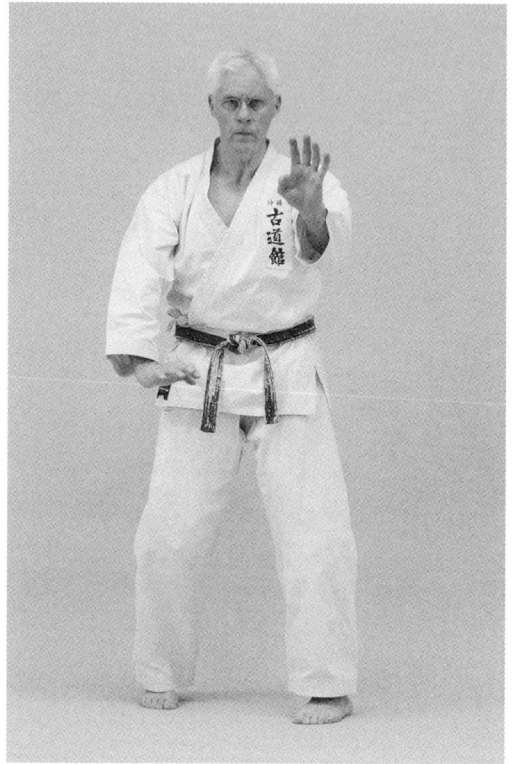

FIGURE 3.57

The right foot steps across, pivoting into a left-foot-forward sanchin dachi facing south. At the same time, the right arm moves in a semicircular counterclockwise motion from outside to inside, ending in the down position. The left arm moves up in a semicircular counterclockwise motion from inside to outside, ending in the upper position (repeating the techniques described in step 43 above). (S—steps 57 through 59)

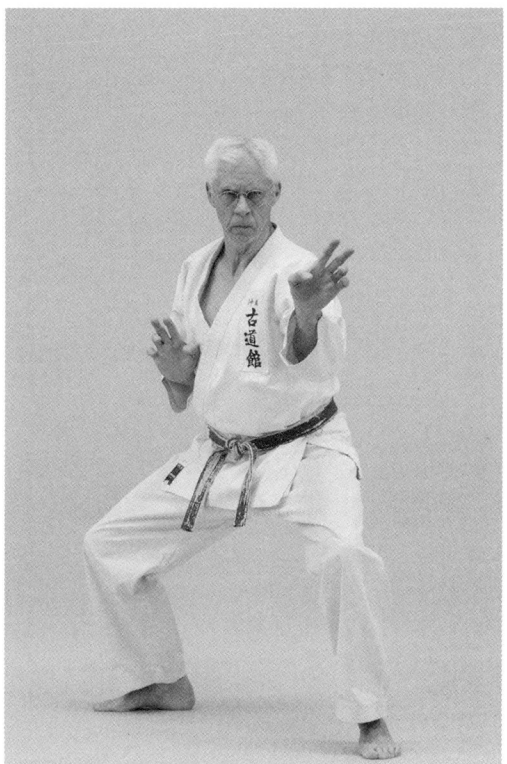

FIGURE 3.58

Shifting forward and dropping into a left-foot-forward shiko dachi, both arms describe slightly offset circular counterclockwise blocking motions, ending with the left arm up, palm forward, and the right arm a bit lower, with the palm facing forward at the center of the chest (see fig. 2.68 for application).

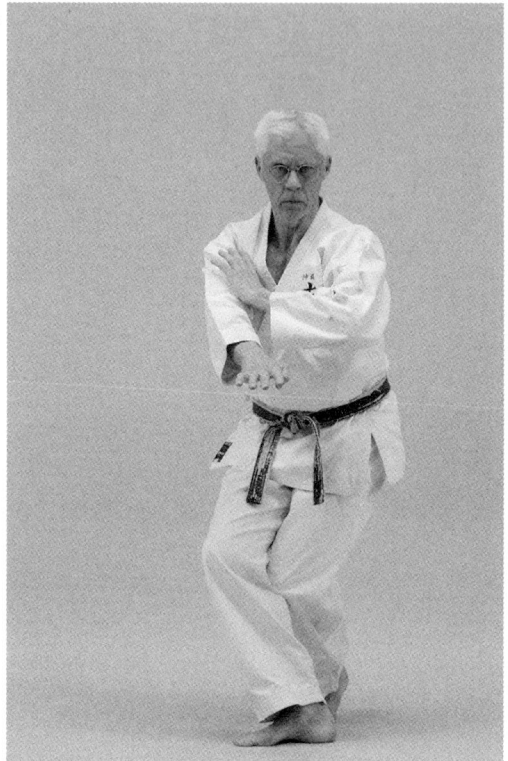

FIGURE 3.59

The right spear hand is thrust under the left arm, with the left hand brought back toward the right shoulder. This is sometimes either accompanied by or followed by a right cross-step—the right foot stepping over the left foot (see fig. 2.69 for application). Some schools will omit this step and simply execute the right spear hand without a step. It all depends on the distance of the defender from the opponent and the space one might need to execute the final technique.

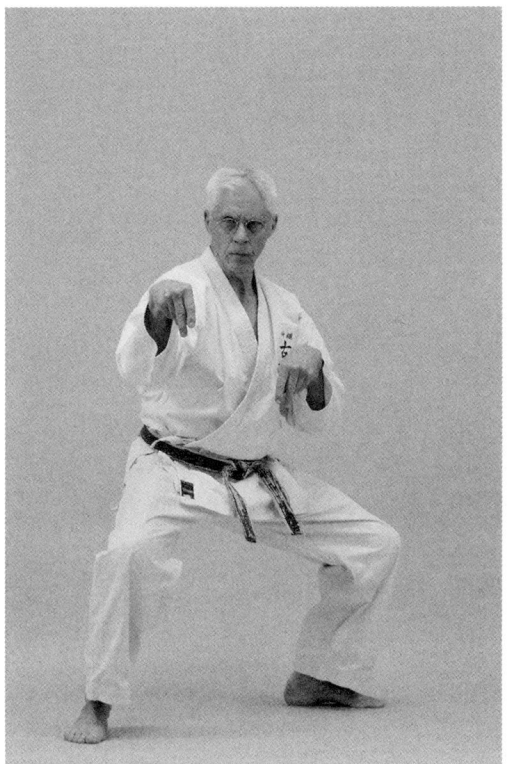

FIGURE 3.60

Stepping across with the left foot into a right-foot-forward shiko dachi facing the original front (N), the hands circle in front of the chest, ending in the bent wrist posture. How exactly the hands circle varies considerably from school to school, and in any case it is difficult to illustrate with still photographs. The hands finish, however, with the left hand, fingers pointing down, at the center of the chest, and the right hand, fingers pointing down, in front at shoulder height. (N—steps 60 through 63)

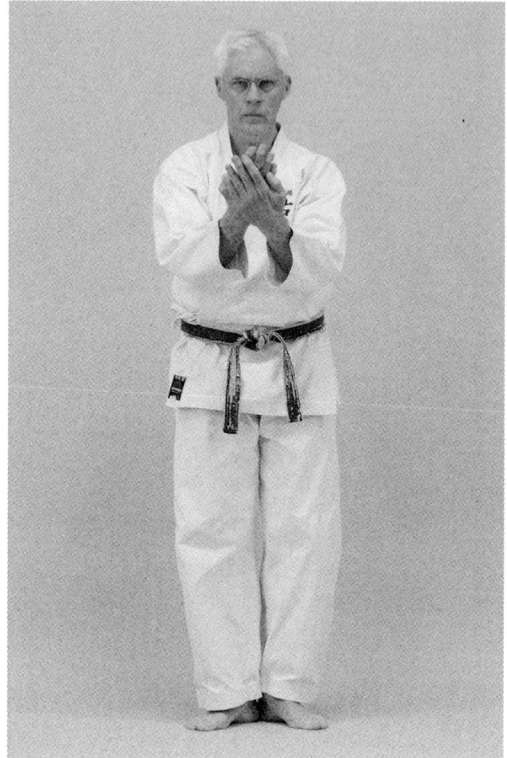

FIGURE 3.61

The right foot is drawn back, meeting the left foot in musubi dachi, as the hands are brought together, left palm pressing on the back of the right hand. This position looks the same as step 2 above.

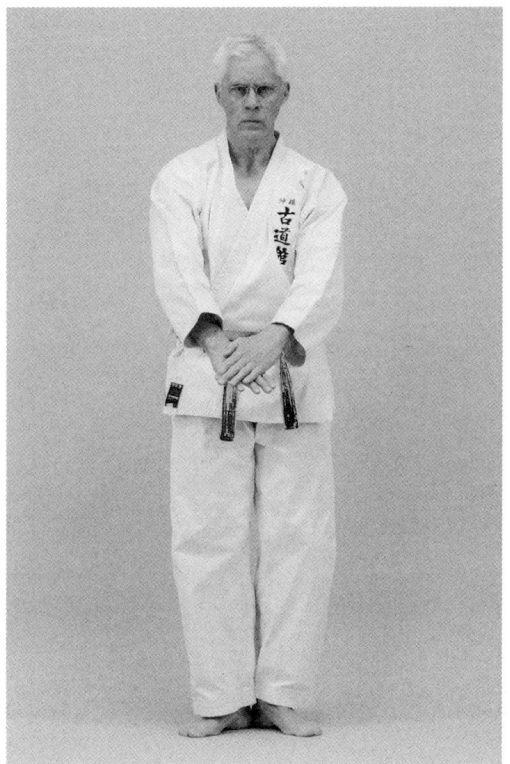

FIGURE 3.62

The hands are then lowered and held for the count of three breaths, each deeper and slower, until the breath is settled. This position is the same as step 3 above.

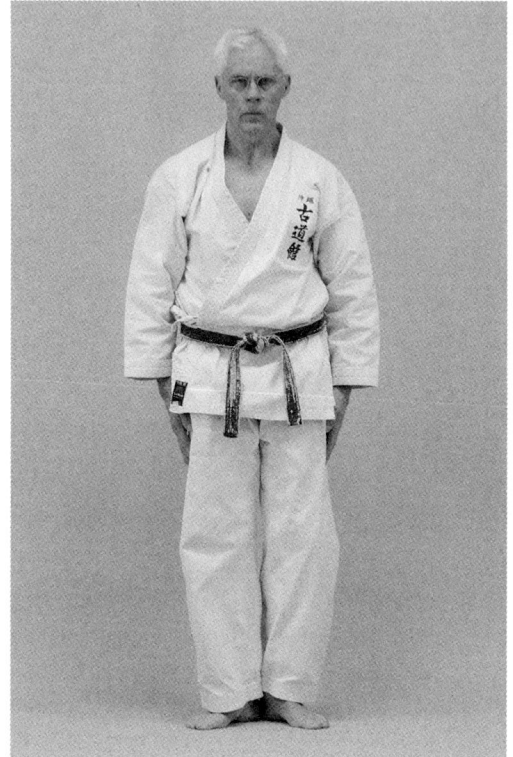

FIGURE 3.63

At the finish of the kata, the hands are brought to the sides, finishing in the same musubi dachi attention stance that begins the kata.

Afterword

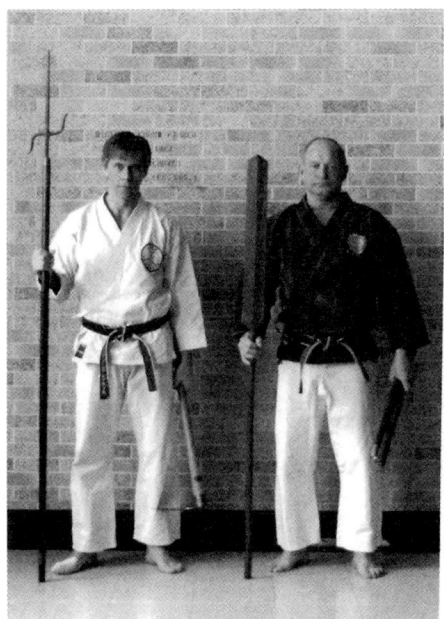

The author with Kimo Wall sensei.

I FIRST MET KIMO SENSEI in the early 1980s. He had come up from Puerto Rico to teach at the University of Massachusetts Amherst at the end of the school year. His old student, Dionisio Perez, was graduating and returning to Puerto Rico at the end of the semester. Kimo sensei came up to take over the karate club that Dionisio had started. The second semester of that first year, Kimo sensei taught *kobudo*, the ancient weapons art of Okinawa.

Sensei had put a small ad in the college newspaper advertising a weapons class at the university. By chance, I saw the ad and showed up at the classroom for an initial information session and a chance to meet "Kimo Wall." At the time, I didn't even know what sort of name Kimo was or what to expect.

I was both taken aback and pleasantly surprised. A gentleman dressed in a sport coat and short brim hat stuck out his hand and introduced himself, "Hello, I'm Kimo." I had been used to an entirely different breed of martial arts instructors, ones whose arrogance was always on display and who spoke pidgin English. Here was a friendly, personable, and outgoing teacher, one who, I would later learn, was also quite willing to explain everything that he taught.

That first semester of training at the university was a kobudo intensive. We trained for two hours every day, and Sensei taught the four base weapons of the Matayoshi kobudo system: the bo, *sai, tonfa,* and *nunchiyaku.* We generally worked out for about an hour and a half, and then Sensei would grab a chair and, as we sat on the floor of the big gym, he would tell stories of Matayoshi sensei and training in Okinawa. He taught us how to fold a gi and tie a belt, the formalities of a traditional Okinawan dojo, and also how to take care of our weapons. He told us stories of how Matayoshi sensei would send them out into the fields to learn how a *kama* was really used or how they used to make a rokushaku bo from a piece of wood scraped down with the broken shard of a Coca-Cola bottle. He showed us how to cut down the handle of a tonfa and shorten the middle section of a *sansetsukon.* He taught us how to string the nunchiyaku and wrap the handle of the sai. But most of the time, he just asked if anyone had any questions, and then the stories grew out of that.

At some point that summer, Kimo sensei and I started to hang out and spend more time together outside of training. I had been training different martial arts for about ten years by this time, and I was also a bit older than most of the students who came to train, so I suppose it was natural that we would become good friends. Yet I always looked at him first and foremost as my teacher.

One afternoon, Sensei said he wanted to show me a karate kata. Up to this point, I had only trained kobudo with him, learning kata for each of the four base weapons and also acting as his uke or fall guy for the weapons kumite we did at demonstrations. But that afternoon, I followed Sensei through Suparinpei. This was my introduction to Goju-ryu. At the time, I didn't know any other kata of the system. As was Sensei's usual instruction model, we walked through the kata three times. Once it seemed as though I remembered the order of the techniques reasonably well, I was on my own. From there, it was, for the most part, a matter of observation and practice. Occasionally, Sensei would watch as I did the kata, making corrections where there was an obvious mistake, but he never over-corrected, realizing that a lot of mistakes take care of themselves over time.

I've always thought it a bit curious that I essentially learned Goju-ryu backwards, starting with Suparinpei. I'll never really know why he did that. He had never done it before, and I don't believe he ever did it again with anyone else. So I've known Suparinpei kata—that is, I've been able to make my way through the sequences of the kata—for almost forty years. And it has taken me almost that long to understand it.

Of course, in any kata there may still be a certain amount of ambiguity. And perhaps we should expect that to be the case, since kata only shows us one side of a confrontation. Exactly how one twists the head in the series of shiko dachi angle techniques at the beginning of the kata is one example of this ambiguity. Why the second complete sequence seems to show two, or even three, different possible endings is another. But we should remember that this sort of ambiguity, whether it's intentional or not, and limited as it is, should not be a license for wild speculation or an endorsement of the view that kata techniques have multiple interpretations, fertile ground for the martial imagination. In most cases with the classical subjects, this ambiguity is really a question of how certain techniques are meant to be applied or how we should understand the structure of a given kata, not the techniques themselves.

Notwithstanding these occasional ambiguities, however, I have come to believe that Suparinpei is the key to understanding so much else in Goju-ryu. This, in fact, is one of the reasons I think it's important to share the lessons I have learned—both the things I am certain of and the questions I still have—after many years of practicing this kata and its bunkai, in front of my teachers and with indispensable training partners. After all, real research, as Kimo sensei often reminded me, takes place on the dojo floor.

Ganbatte kudasai,
Giles Hopkins
June 2019

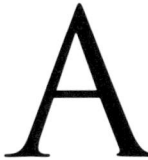

A
THEMATIC CONNECTIONS

THERE IS A THEMATIC CONNECTION not only between the techniques and sequences of a given kata in the classical canon of Goju-ryu but also between the techniques and sequences of different kata within the same system. In fact, this is one of the reasons we can look at it as a system and not just a random collection of kata and techniques. It is also, I would argue, why it is important to study the whole system, because we can find these thematic connections everywhere, not just between Suparinpei, Seisan, and Sanseiru—similarities that have already been pointed out. These thematic similarities often show us variations in how similar techniques are applied, thereby reinforcing our interpretations of specific techniques in any given kata and our understanding of the martial principles involved.

The fact that there are so many obvious thematic connections is probably due in part at least to the general admonition that one should block the arms of the opponent but attack the head. The classical kata illustrate self-defense scenarios for life-threatening confrontations, and so all of the sequences end with an attack to the opponent's head or neck. Most of the time, this means a head-twisting technique that begins with one of the defender's hands controlling the opponent's chin and the other hand on the opponent's head or grabbing the hair, as we see in the sequences of Suparinpei kata.

Sometimes the sequences of kata will show the defender moving into this controlling position almost immediately, as part of the initial receiving technique, and sometimes the defender moves into this position as part of the bridging technique or finishing technique at the end of a sequence. And, since it is so prevalent in the classical subjects of

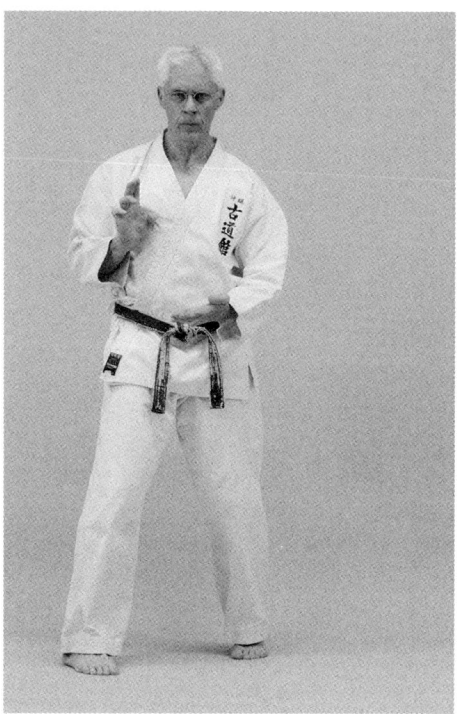

FIGURE A.1

The end position of the mawashi uke and nukite/shuto position from the first half of Suparinpei.

Goju-ryu, it is perhaps a good place to begin if one is studying the thematic connections we see in kata or practicing how to move from one technique to another from a different sequence, which one might do depending on the exigencies of the situation. This is, I believe, an important aspect of one's training.

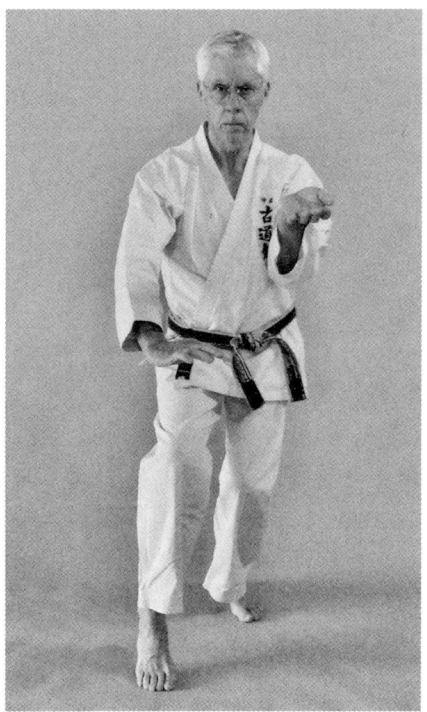

FIGURE A.2

Moving from the mawashi uke and nukite/shuto into the end of the first sequence in Saifa kata. The first step twists the opponent's head while executing a right hiza geri (knee kick).

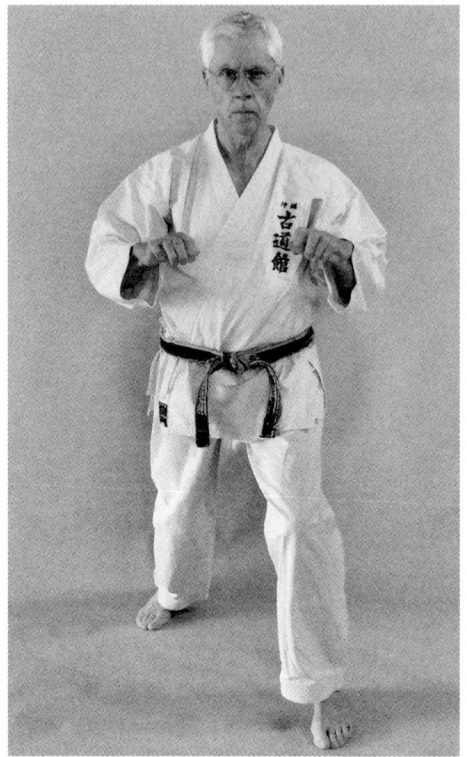

FIGURE A.3

The kick is followed by a pulling-down technique, where the "half fist" is used to pull the opponent down from behind onto the front knee. The curled fingers of the "half fist" show the defender digging into the opponent's trapezius muscles.

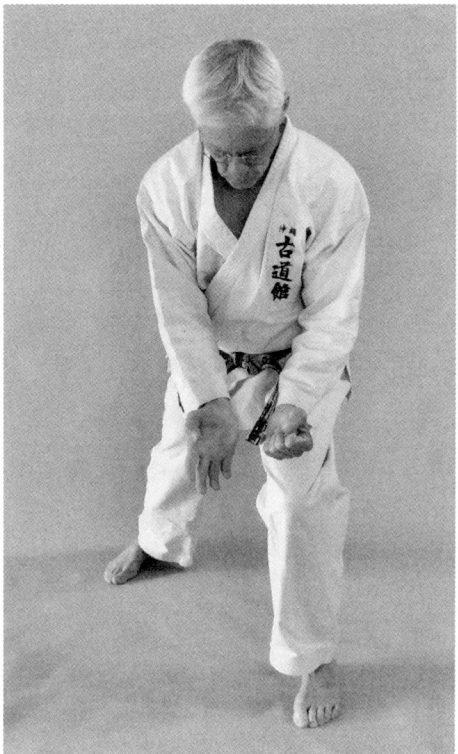

FIGURE A.4

The defender then twists the attacker's head, holding onto the hair, and attacks with a shuto uchi to the throat.

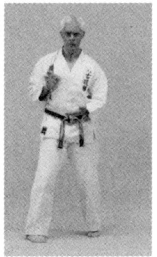 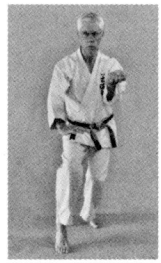 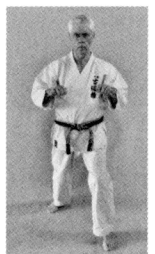 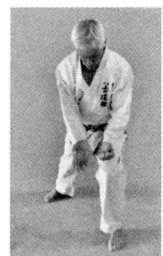

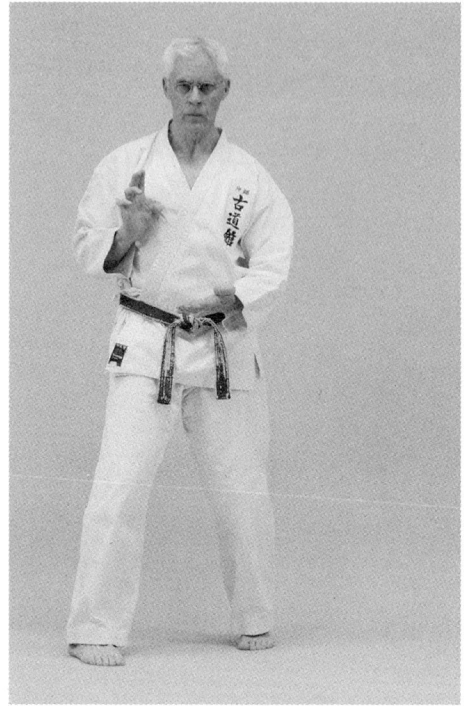

FIGURE A.5

The end position of the mawashi uke and nukite/shuto position from the first half of Suparinpei.

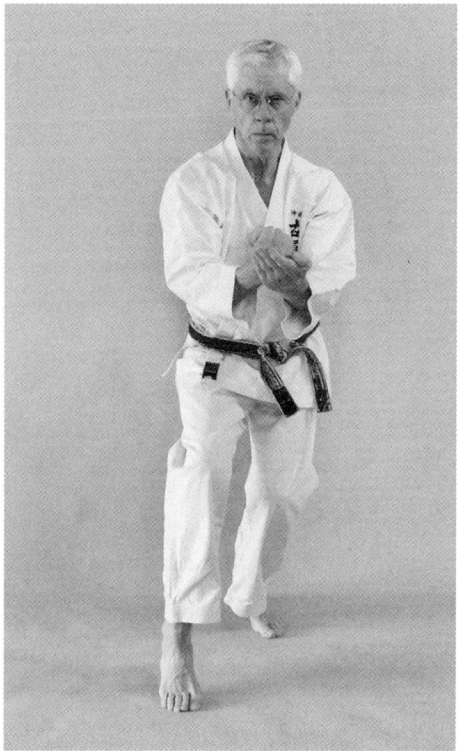

FIGURE A.6

Moving from the mawashi uke and nukite/shuto into the end of the first sequence in Seiunchin kata. Shifting to the side into a right-foot-forward Cat Stance, the right hand holds the attacker's hair and twists the head, moving the attacker.

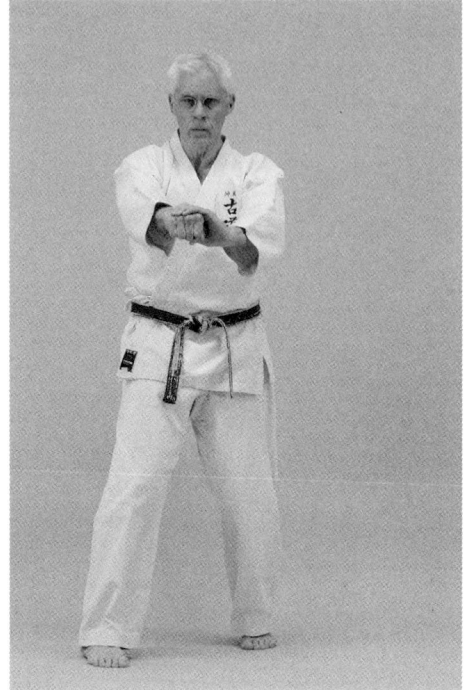

FIGURE A.7

Shifting forward into a right-foot-forward Basic Stance with what has conventionally been described as a "supported punch," the attacker is turned around. The left hand is holding the opponent's chin and the right hand is holding the hair.

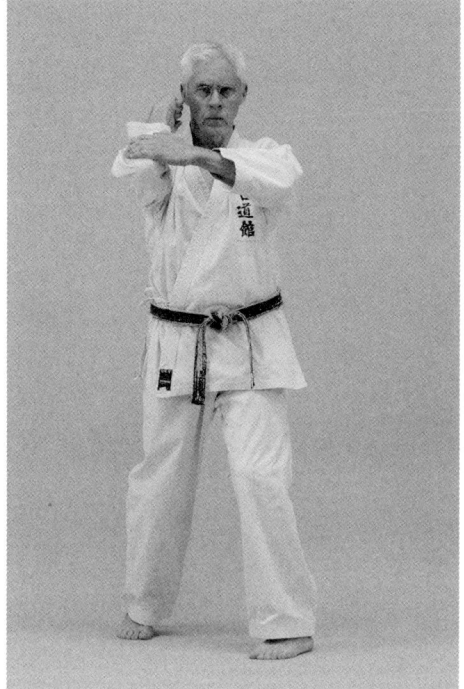

FIGURE A.8

Stepping back into a left-foot-forward Basic Stance, the defender attacks with the right elbow.

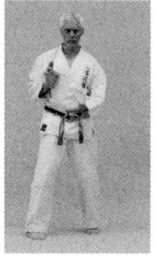 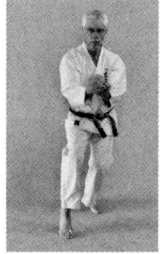 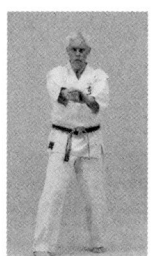 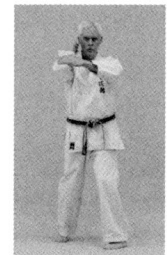

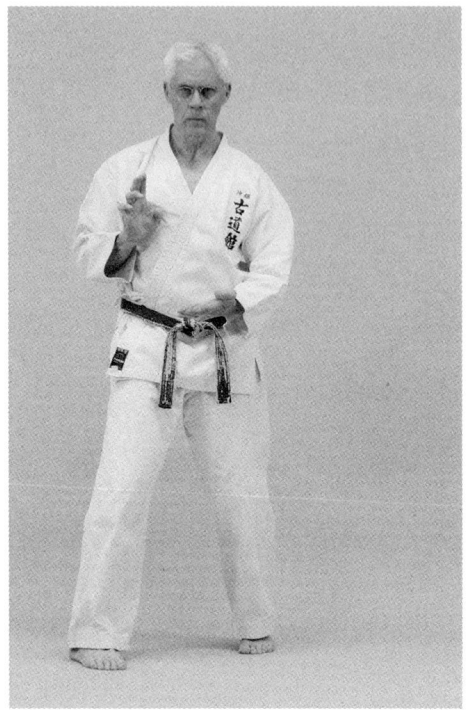

FIGURE A.9

The end position of the mawashi uke and nukite/shuto position from the first half of Suparinpei.

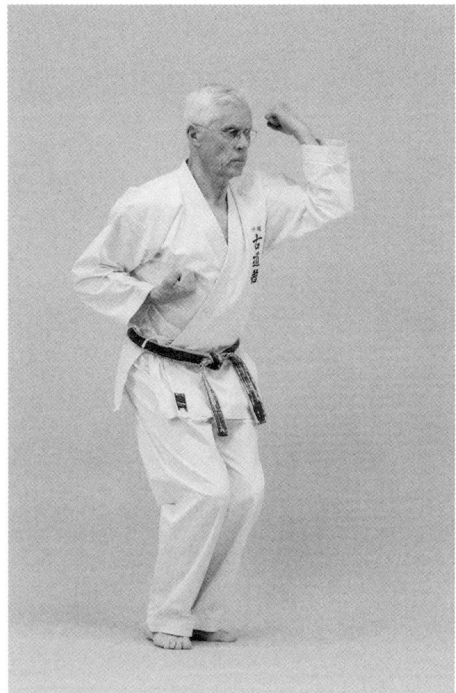

FIGURE A.10

Moving from the mawashi uke and nukite/shuto position into the fin-ishing technique of the first sequence of Shisochin kata, where the left hand of the nukite/shuto pushes the attacker's chin up as the right hand pulls down on the attacker's head or hair, as the defender's feet are brought together, turning to the right at a 90-degree angle to the attacker as the technique is executed.

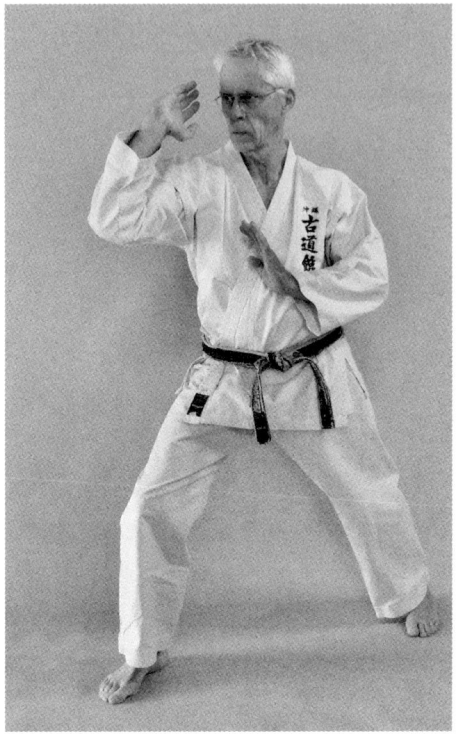

FIGURE A.11

Continuing with techniques from another of the sequences in Shiso-chin, as the defender again turns to the right (clockwise) into a right Front Stance at a 90-degree angle to the attacker, the hands change. With the left hand now on the attacker's head, the right open hand is brought up into the opponent's chin, twisting the head.

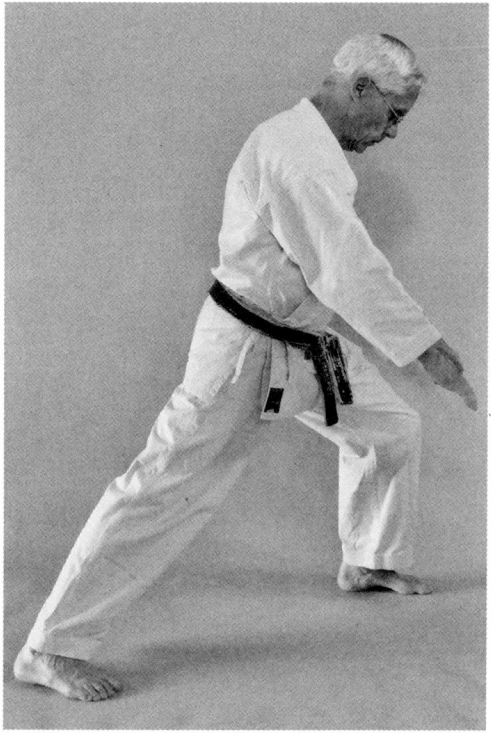

FIGURE A.12

As the defender turns 180 degrees (counterclockwise), the attacker is thrown down onto the defender's front knee. This finishing technique occurs in the middle sequence of the Shodokan (Higa) version of Shisochin kata.

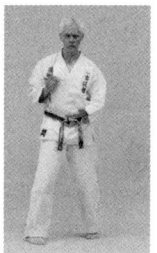 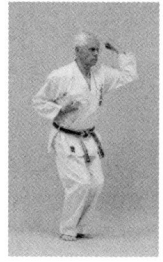 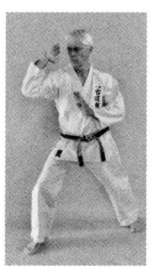 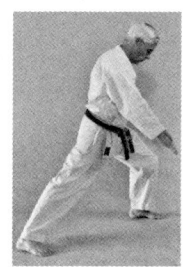

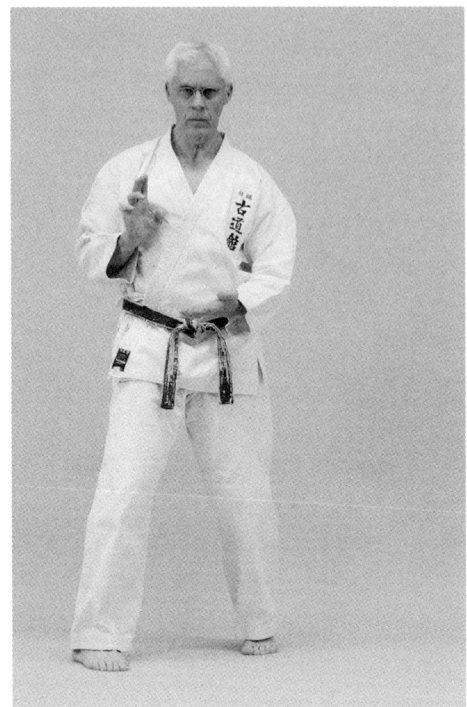

FIGURE A.13

The end position of the mawashi uke and nukite/shuto position from the first half of Suparinpei.

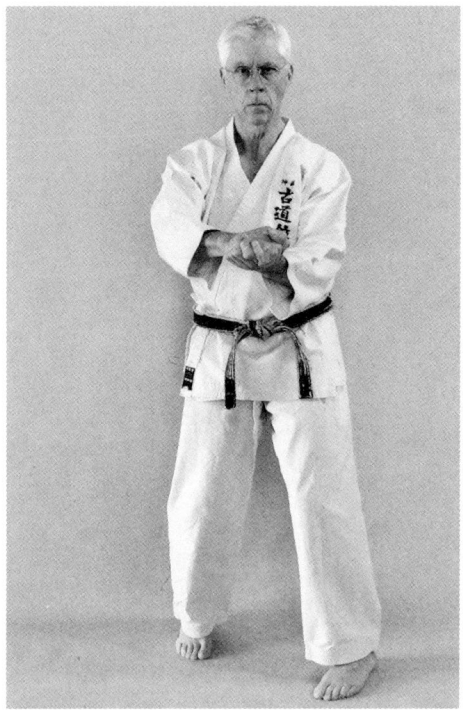

FIGURE A.14

Moving from the mawashi uke and nukite/shuto position into the finishing technique of the first sequence of Seipai kata, where the left open hand, palm up, is brought into the right open hand, palm down. This is the position after the opening technique of Seipai, where the right hand is on top of the opponent's head, and the left hand comes under to grasp the opponent's chin.

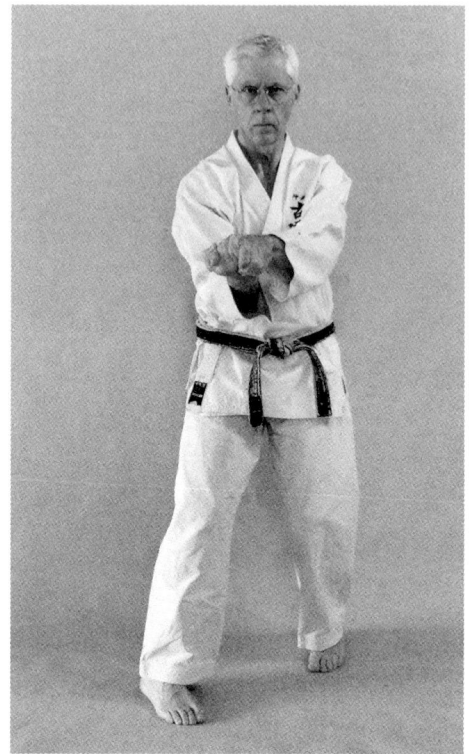

FIGURE A.15

The clasped hands turn over, twisting the opponent's head.

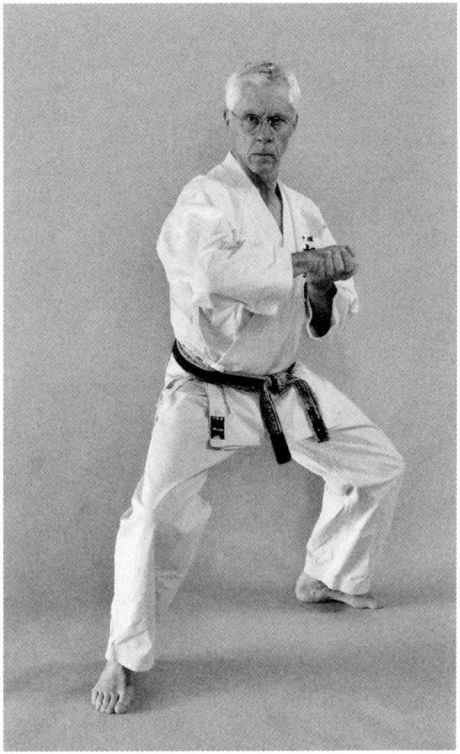

FIGURE A.16

Dropping into shiko dachi, the attacker's head is twisted forcefully. And depending on how one executes the head twist, a hand change is sometimes employed.

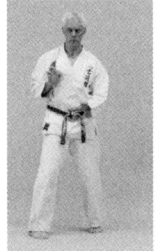 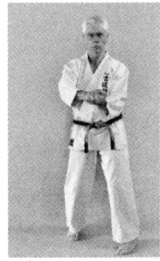 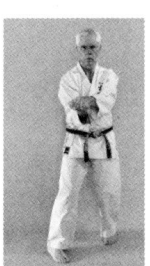 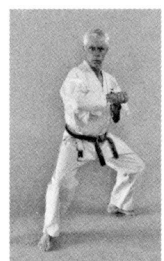

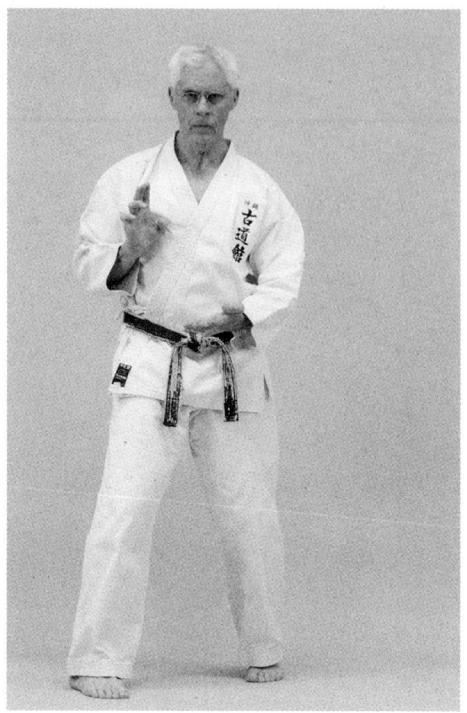

FIGURE A.17

The end position of the mawashi uke and nukite/shuto position from the first half of Suparinpei.

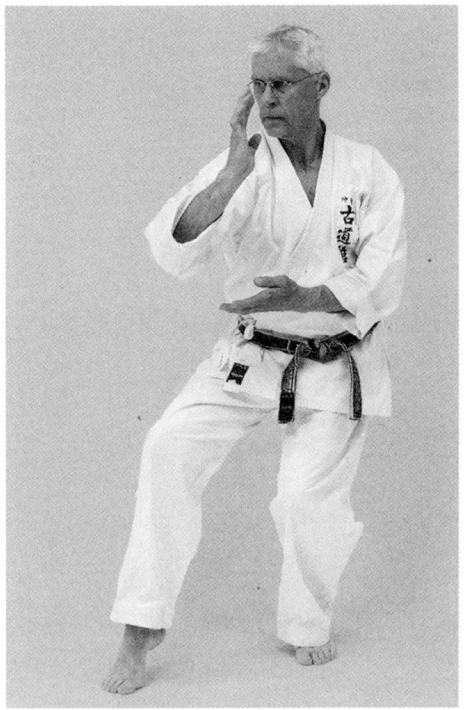

FIGURE A.18

Moving from the mawashi uke and nukite/shuto position into one of the first techniques of Kururunfa by shifting into a right-foot-forward Cat Stance in order to attack with the knee and down side kick combination. The right hand is on the opponent's head.

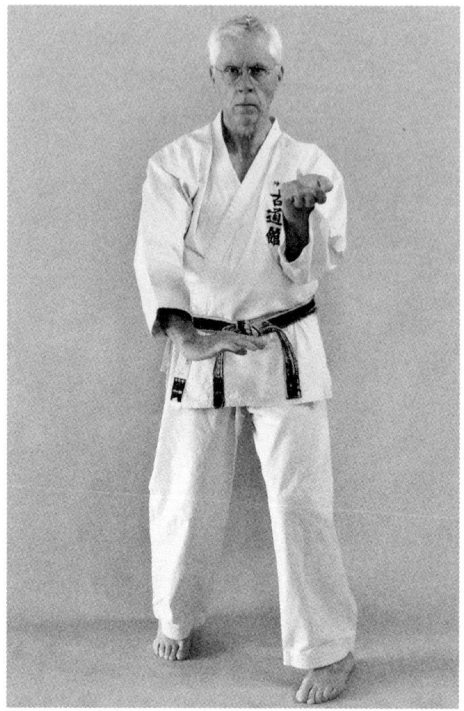

FIGURE A.19

Stepping forward into one of the signature moves of Kururunfa, occurring repeatedly in the opening sequence, the left open hand is brought up into the opponent's chin, as the right hand pulls or pushes down on the opponent's head.

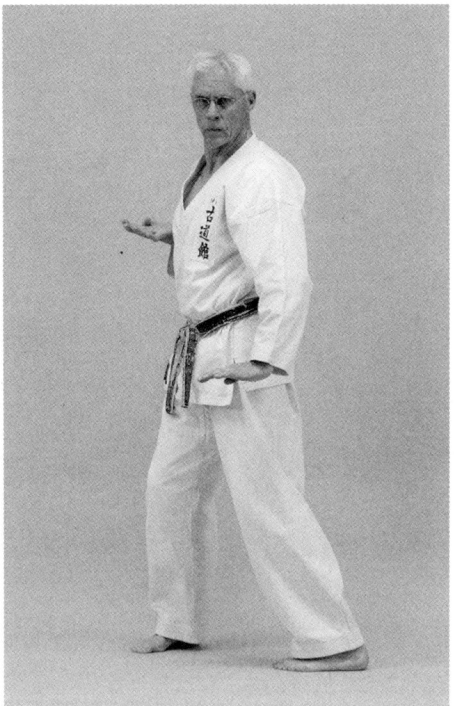

FIGURE A.20

Then, continuing to twist the attacker's head, the defender pivots to throw the attacker to the ground.

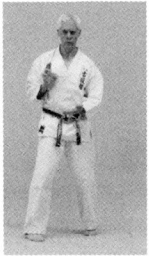 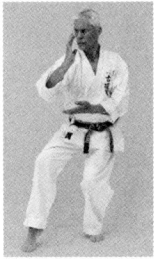 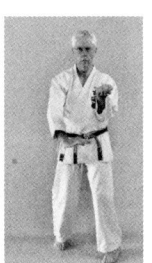 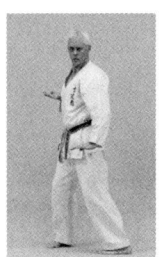

B

KEY POINTS TO REMEMBER IN THE ANALYSIS OF SUPARINPEI KATA

1. Suparinpei is a kata that illustrates close-in fighting strategies. This is indicated by the double-arm kamae posture that begins the kata. This idea is reinforced in Sanseiru and Seisan.

2. Suparinpei kata is composed of two distinct parts, each of which differs in structure. The first half comprises techniques that move to the *outside* of the opponent's defensive posture (with the possible exception of the two-arm spreading technique that follows the initial "punches"). The second half comprises techniques that move to the *inside* of the opponent's defensive posture.

3. Though the double-arm kamae that utilizes the "punch" and retraction may be seen as the first receiving technique in Suparinpei (paired with the double-arm spreading technique), the mawashi uke and nukite/shuto is the receiving technique that introduces each of the three series of finishing techniques that make up the bulk of the first half of the kata. The mawashi in Cat Stance, the double punch, and the angular shiko dachi techniques are each meant to be connected to the initial mawashi uke to form a complete application sequence. The double punch and angular shiko dachi techniques,

as we see them performed in kata, come off the opposite side (left) mawashi uke and nukite/shuto.

4. The second half of Suparinpei comprises three complete bunkai sequences. Each sequence begins with the same blocking or receiving technique—that is, each arm moving in a semicircular sweeping block against the opponent's arms. These entry techniques are also seen in each of the three complete sequences of Seisan kata. In addition to the initial receiving techniques, each sequence comprises bridging or controlling techniques and finishing techniques.

5. The second complete bunkai sequence of the second half shows two alternate finishes: the sweeping crescent kick and the jumping kick and head twist.

6. There are two kinds of mawashi techniques: the mawashi uke in Basic Stance, a *receiving* technique, shown in Suparinpei with the nukite/shuto technique, and the mawashi in Cat Stance, a *finishing* technique used to twist the opponent's head and attack with the front knee. Both of these mawashi techniques are shown in Suparinpei kata. The mawashi uke in Basic Stance only occurs in one other kata of Goju-ryu—Sanchin. The finishing mawashi in Cat Stance, however, occurs in a number of other kata.

7. Each of the sequences of Suparinpei finishes with a head-twisting or neck-breaking technique. This is true of the first half techniques and the second half sequences, and, of course, what we find in the sequences of each of the other classical kata also. Generally speaking, in Goju-ryu we block the arms, but attack the head.

8. In Suparinpei kata, the change in direction we see in the second half of the kata usually indicates the beginning of a new sequence. Directional changes in some kata may indicate moving off line or, in more colloquial terms, getting out of the way. The techniques of Suparinpei are generally for close combat—confrontations that either begin from a clinch or grappling position or quickly devolve into one. However, the techniques we see in the first half

of the kata—indicated by the 90- and 180-degree turns—generally necessitate directional changes in order to effectively employ the techniques.

9. The sun and moon block that we see in the Higa or Shodokan version of Seisan figures prominently in Suparinpei. This is just one of the connections that we see between Suparinpei, Seisan, Sanseiru, and Sanchin. An understanding of the techniques of Suparinpei will help one to see similarities and variations in the other classical kata as well, but these four kata clearly exhibit an especially strong link. Most of the techniques one sees in Seisan and Sanseiru can be found in Suparinpei in one form or another. And these connections will help to reinforce one's interpretation and analysis of kata techniques.

10. The inside forearm technique that we see in the second and third complete sequences of the second half of Suparinpei is an important bridging or controlling technique in Seisan, Kururunfa, and Shisochin as well. It is generally employed with either forward movement or a turn.

11. Most of the striking that we see in Suparinpei is done with the open hand, in the form of either a shuto or knife-edge attack, as we see in the second complete sequence, or a palm strike, as we see in the last sequence. This is also true of Goju-ryu in general; that is, punching techniques, despite what countless hours of makiwara training would indicate, are actually not very characteristic of the Goju system.

12. Oral history suggests that Miyagi Chojun sensei closed the hand in Kanryo Higashionna sensei's Sanchin kata. This is worth keeping in mind. If the beginning posture of Sanchin that we practice today was originally an open-hand posture, perhaps the same was true of the opening posture—and the initial "punching" techniques—of Sanseiru, Seisan, and Suparinpei. One should keep this in mind when studying the applications of kata.

13. The rhythm we so often see in the performance of kata is usually the same rhythm we use to teach the individual movements—the position of the hands and feet, executed one step at a time in a staccato or stop-action fashion. In application, the movements of any given sequence are fluid and connected. It is difficult to see the applications of a sequence when the movements are performed in the same highly punctuated manner that's used when a kata is first learned. One should keep this in mind when analyzing the techniques of Suparinpei or, in fact, any of the Kaishu kata.

14. Finally, kata movements should not be overly stylized, and unnecessary flourishes should be avoided. Kata performances, even by high-level experienced practitioners, often suffer from both of these tendencies toward showmanship, hindering one's ability to interpret and apply the techniques of the kata. There should be no unnecessary movements in kata.

NOTES

1 Nigel Sutton, *Tai Chi Chuan Roots & Branches* (Clarendon, VT: Tuttle, 2011), 114.

2 Patrick McCarthy, "Kata: The Enigma of Uchinadi," FightingArts.com, August 26, 2001, http://tinyurl.com/y9qaptyr.

3 Patrick McCarthy and Yukio McCarthy, *Ancient Okinawan Martial Arts, Volume 2: Koryu Uchinadi* (Boston: Tuttle, 1999), 51.

4 McCarthy and McCarthy, *Ancient Okinawan Martial Arts*, 65–66.

5 For more on this, see Giles Hopkins, *Wandering Along the Way of Okinawan Karate: Thinking about Goju-Ryu* (Berkeley, CA: Blue Snake Books, 2020).

6 For a more complete explanation, see Hopkins, *Wandering Along the Way of Okinawan Karate*.

7 McCarthy and McCarthy, *Ancient Okinawan Martial Arts*, 53.

8 Giles Hopkins, *The Kata and Bunkai of Goju-Ryu Karate: The Essence of the Heishu and Kaishu Kata* (Berkeley, CA: Blue Snake Books, 2018).

9 For a more in-depth description of this technique, see Hopkins, *The Kata and Bunkai of Goju-Ryu Karate*.

10 For a more complete description of this bunkai, see Hopkins, *The Kata and Bunkai of Goju-Ryu Karate*. And one can only imagine that the hands, working again in opposition, are twisting the opponent's head here also.

11 See Hopkins, *The Kata and Bunkai of Goju-Ryu Karate* for a brief discussion of this technique and some of these interpretations.

INDEX

ABOUT THE AUTHOR

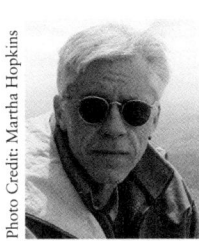

GILES HOPKINS is a longtime karate instructor and the author of a number of magazine articles and books, including *The Kata and Bunkai of Goju-Ryu Karate* and *Wandering Along the Way of Okinawan Karate* (Blue Snake Books). A practitioner of martial arts since 1973, he is a sixth-degree black belt in Okinawan Goju-ryu and a fifth-degree black belt with a teaching certificate in Matayoshi kobudo from the Zen Okinawan Kobudo Renmei.

A retired English teacher with three wonderful grown children, Hopkins lives in Northampton, Massachusetts, with his wife, where he continues to train, teach, and write about the martial arts.

About North Atlantic Books

North Atlantic Books (NAB) is an independent, nonprofit publisher committed to a bold exploration of the relationships between mind, body, spirit, and nature. Founded in 1974, NAB aims to nurture a holistic view of the arts, sciences, humanities, and healing. To make a donation or to learn more about our books, authors, events, and newsletter, please visit www.northatlanticbooks.com.

North Atlantic Books is the publishing arm of the Society for the Study of Native Arts and Sciences, a 501(c)(3) nonprofit educational organization that promotes cross-cultural perspectives linking scientific, social, and artistic fields. To learn how you can support us, please visit our website.